JOURNEY
of the
HEART

a memoir
Richard Crystal

Published in the United States by TitleTown Publishing, LLC
www.titletownpublishing.com

Distributed by Midpoint Trade Books
www.midpointtrade.com

Cover Design: Mark Karis
Interior Layout and Design: Erika L. Block
Cover Photo: Copyright © Jackie Gay Wilson

ISBN 978–0996295-15-4 (hardcover)
Printed in the United States of America

First Edition

Library of Congress Cataloging-in-Publication Data available upon request.

for Jackie

Contents

"Preserve your memories;
They're all that's left you."

—Paul Simon

Foreword

by Kareem Abdul-Jabbar

The passage from adolescence to maturity—from worrying about our hairstyle to worrying about where our hair went—is a journey of ever-increasing challenges. The youthful conviction of our own invulnerability and immortality soon deteriorates into the inevitable tending to our growing list of ailments, some just annoying, some life-threatening. *The Jetsons* promised us Baby Boomers flying cars, robot servants, and a happy, pain-free old age. As I have found out through my quadruple bypass surgery and a diagnosis of leukemia, it ain't necessarily so.

The poet Stanislaw Jerzy Lec once wrote, "Youth is the gift of nature, but age is a work of art." The emphasis is on the word "work," because that's what aging requires: hard work. But, as I discovered from reading Richard's invaluable book, it also requires good humor, self-searching, and an awareness that we're not in this alone. In his book, Richard discusses the issues of his health with humor, candor, and wisdom, thereby making it a lot easier for the rest of us who have to walk his same path. As Richard points out, it's a journey that can be scary and threatening, but it also can be fulfilling and rewarding. We are fortunate to have Richard to illuminate that path for us.

Preface

In the fall of 2008, I had breakfast with Steven Cagan, a gifted composer and my friend of over thirty years. He had recently introduced me to "The Tender Bar," J.R. Moehringer's wonderful memoir about growing up on Long Island in the seventies. As I thanked him for the great read, he added that he hoped the book would inspire me to consider writing my own memoir. Granted, I had once sold an article about the riots at the Newport Jazz Festival to High Fidelity Magazine in 1971 and had minor success as a Hollywood screenwriter, but this was something else entirely. I laughed at the presumptuous suggestion, feeling that it was a premature notion. Further, the thought was intimidating for I was quite certain I didn't have the literary chops to confront such a challenge.

About a month later, on a nearby golf course in Encino, I experienced a rapid heartbeat and a burning in my chest whenever I would push my cart uphill. I immediately saw my cardiologist, who informed me that I needed to have open heart surgery to replace my aortic valve. We discussed potential options, but I really didn't have any. If I refused to undergo the procedure, I would most probably be dead from a massive heart attack within three years.

The sobering reality of my condition put me face to face with my mortality. Unexpected waves of emotion swept over me. My wife, Fran, gave me a journal to record the unfolding events of my surgery and to serve as an outlet for my feelings. And so I began to keep a diary. There were notes, times, images, even a poem or two. But nothing more.

When I began to regain my strength after the surgery, I found myself re-reading my journal and exploring some of my notes in greater detail. It began to intrigue me. What was really underneath these momentary images that popped into my head?

About a month into my recovery, I saw my cardiologist, Dr. Ilan Kedan, for a follow up. On my way out of his office, he asked me if I had gotten back to writing again. I told him I had. In fact, I was actually writing about the heart surgery. Dr. Kedan thought it was a wonderful idea and expressed interest in reading the finished work. It could be a helpful tool for his patients who would be undergoing a similar procedure.

It was the encouragement I needed.

I began to take the project seriously and started writing every day. I envisioned a short pamphlet for heart patients that would serve as a helpful aid, an honest account of the process. Using the notes in my journal as a launching pad, I began to recall, in great detail, the chain of events that began with my episode on the golf course. But as I continued working, something else began to emerge. The surgery that had opened my chest had unlocked a flood of memories. Like an archaeologist uncovering a buried city, I began to dig deeper and deeper and slowly rediscovered the events that had shaped my life.

Prologue

It was a beautiful day.

I stood on the first tee and looked down the fairway one last time before taking my back swing. I approached the ball, did a little waggle in the hopes of keeping loose, and repeated the mantra in my head, "You don't play golf to relax, you relax to play golf." The head of the driver came down and made contact. Ping!

I lifted my head and watched with relief as the ball flew into the air and landed just off the left side of the fairway.

"Good hit, Rip," Sandy shouted in encouragement.

"I'll take it," I replied.

I put the driver in my golf bag and started wheeling my cart down the fairway to take my next shot. I love to walk the eighteen holes. Even if I play like a hack, I can always take comfort in the fact that I get great exercise. As I pushed my cart up a small hill on the way to my ball, I felt a slight burning in my chest. I reached up nonchalantly and started rubbing it.

"You okay?" Sandy asked.

"Yeah, I'm okay. Just got this burning going on. Feels like some kind of indigestion."

"I get it too. It's probably acid reflux. Pop a Zantac before a round, and you'll be fine."

Sandy's diagnosis made perfect sense, and, by the time I reached my ball, the burning had all but disappeared. Feeling like my normal self again, my focus returned to the challenge confronting me for my next shot. I was about a hundred and forty yards away from the pin on the short par four. The seven iron felt right. Definitely a seven iron. I stood over the ball, reminding myself to keep my head down and follow through. Don't try to kill it. You've got plenty of club.

I started my back swing, trying to feel the right tempo, turned my shoulder, came down with my club, and made solid contact. The ball lifted high into the air and landed on the front end of the green. Awesome. Now all I had to do to get my par was two putt.

The first putt was crucial. I needed to get the ball within three feet of the hole to seal the deal. I studied the green and saw that it was basically straight – very little break, if any. That was a good thing. Just keep that head down, putt through the ball, and I should be okay. My stroke was steady, and the ball had a nice roll to it. My eyes widened with hopeful expectation as the dimpled white orb approached the hole. It slid by the right side of the cup at the very last moment, but I was only slightly disappointed. I'm a bogey golfer and a birdie is a rare occurrence. Hell, I'll take a tap-in regulation par any time. Any time at all.

Ah, yes. What a lovely way to start the round.

As I lined up my drive on the second hole, I felt a surge of positive energy. This was going to be my day. Filled with confidence, I took a bigger backswing than usual. I watched with dismay as the ball hooked into the rough on the right side of the fairway. I shook my head. What a humbling game. The moment you think you've figured it out, it slaps you back into reality. As I started pushing my cart up the steep incline towards my ball, I suddenly felt the burning in my chest again. I guess my indigestion wasn't gone after all. But as soon as I found myself on level ground, the burning in my chest magically disappeared.

As I continued playing the front nine, this pattern repeated itself again and again. I started to grow concerned. After I teed off on the tenth hole, things really got freaky. My heart suddenly started beating rapidly. I'd felt that sensation before and expected my heart to slow down in a few minutes.

It didn't.

My heart raced for almost an hour. And, when it finally calmed down, I felt exhausted. Something was definitely wrong. What the hell was going on?

Chapter One
The Time Has Come

I was startled from a deep sleep by the grating buzz of my alarm. I groped in the morning darkness for the clock on my night stand and quickly shut it off. In fifteen minutes, it would be six a.m. My kid brother, Billy, rolled over in bed and wrapped the blanket tightly around him. It was a cold fall morning. I threw on a pair of worn out jeans, a hooded sweatshirt, and laced up my black converse sneakers. I tip-toed past the door to my parent's bedroom, making sure I didn't make a sound. My dad had gotten home from working in the city a few hours earlier, and there would be hell to pay if I woke him up. I continued down the narrow hallway, past the small bedroom where my older brother Joel slept on the high riser under the open window on the side of our tiny house. I moved quickly past the kitchen a few feet away. Breakfast would have to wait until later. I didn't want to be late. I threw on a windbreaker that hung on a hook in the front closet and headed out the front door to the street. I hung a left, broke into a sprint, and made it to the nearby Cozy Nook in record time.

Julie Kantor, the owner of the neighborhood luncheonette on East Park Avenue, was just opening the front door. The stacks of Sunday papers were piled high, dropped off in the middle of the night by the news trucks that made the forty-five minute trip from Manhattan.

"Hey, kid, how you doin'?" Julie said with a sense of relief.

"Good morning, Julie," I replied.

Julie held the door open for me as I made my way inside. I grabbed the hand dolly in front of the magazine rack and wheeled it back outside. Just five hours before, my fingers blackened from the fresh print, I was putting the Saturday night edition together for local customers that couldn't wait to get it home. I began stacking the bundled papers from the street onto the dolly. After a number of trips, when everything was moved inside, I sliced the metal bindings with wire cutters and collated the morning edition with the rest of the paper I had put together the day before.

Fifty years ago, in 1959, newspapers in New York were a big deal. You could read all about it in the pages of the New York Times, the Herald Tribune, the Journal American, the Daily News, and the Daily Mirror. There were only three television networks at the time, no CNN, no internet, no cellphones or faxes. If you wanted to know what was happening in the world, you read the paper. And that's what people did.

For the next four hours, until about ten in the morning, I would put the Sunday papers together. When my work was done, I'd stagger to the counter in a mild state of exhaustion and collapse on a swivel seat. Chico, the short order cook, would wink and pour me a hot cup of coffee, then smile as he watched me devour a huge breakfast of bacon and eggs that he made for me.

We never had a lot of money. Just got by. Going out to eat at a local restaurant was a rare event. Spending a Christmas vacation in Miami Beach was only a dream. Sleep away camp – not a chance. I never, ever had an allowance. If I wanted spending money, I had to earn it. I babysat, collected wagons in the parking lot at the local supermarket, worked as a beachcomber, and even put the Sunday papers together at the Cozy Nook. But that was fine with me for there was no better feeling than having Julie Kantor reach into the cash register and hand me that ten dollar bill when the job was finished. I took great pride in knowing that I earned every bit of that money and could spend it in any way I saw fit.

My name is Richard, but everyone calls me Rip.

I was the second of three sons born to Jack and Helen Crystal some sixty-three years ago at the Fifth Avenue Hospital in New York City. In 1950, when I was four years old, our family joined the mass exodus from the concrete jungle to the greener pastures of the exploding nearby suburbs. We settled in the small seaside community of Long Beach on the south shore of Long Island because my grandmother was ill and her doctor thought the salty air would be therapeutic.

Long Beach turned out to be a great place to grow up.

Everyone who lived there was part of an extended family. Doors were always unlocked, and, if you were in the neighborhood, you'd drop by a friend's home and say hello. You never thought you were intruding.

You always felt welcome. If you needed to get someplace fast, you'd put your thumb out on Park Avenue and, within minutes, a car would stop, a neighbor would open the door, and give you a lift. I thrived in Long Beach. Life was pretty darn good. But nothing lasts forever.

Everything suddenly changed with an unexpected phone call from my mom in the fall of 1963, during my first semester at the University of Bridgeport. I sat in stunned disbelief as she struggled to tell me that my father had died of a massive heart attack in a local bowling alley. He was just fifty-four. A month later, President Kennedy was shot down in Dallas.

I would never be the same.

I lived through the turmoil of the sixties – the civil rights movement, the war in Vietnam, the assassinations of RFK and Martin Luther King, Jr. I smoked pot, read Carlos Castaneda, dropped acid a couple of times, slept with a lot of women, and taught myself how to play guitar. As the seventies began, I struggled to find my path. I tried forging a career as an accountant, a lawyer, a teacher, a jewelry salesman, and a theatrical agent. There were a lot of bumps and pitfalls along the way, but I continued to believe that somehow, some way, everything was going to be okay.

For most of my life, I have been blessed with good health. During my years at Long Beach High School, I was the point guard on my basketball team and pitched and played first base on the baseball team. I took up long distance running in my early thirties, logging three to five miles a day for almost twenty years. I never was a smoker, watched what I ate, and had an annual physical to keep an eye on any signs of trouble.

During one of these once a year visits about fifteen years ago, my doctor put a stethoscope on my chest, listened to my heart, and detected a murmur. He immediately referred me to a cardiologist to find out what was causing it. The source of my murmur was a bicuspid aortic valve – a congenital abnormality. The valve had two flaps instead of the normal three and didn't shut properly. As a result, my heart was working harder to distribute my blood throughout my body. My cardiologist informed me that the day would come when my valve would have to be replaced.

I shook my head in disbelief. I felt great. No one had more energy than I did. I vowed to continue to take care of myself and, in doing so, would prove him wrong. I exercised daily, did stretches, worked with light weights. At the age of fifty, I took up golf and walked the eighteen holes whenever I could. The years passed by and I continued to feel great. I kept a keen eye on my health with an annual checkup and diligently monitored my heart. Perhaps I wouldn't need a new valve after all. As Dr. Kedan studied my echocardiogram, a test in which ultrasound is used to examine the heart, he shook his head and uttered the words that would dramatically change my life: "I think it's time."

I met Dr. Kedan at my annual heart exam the year before. Like my previous cardiologist, Dr. Kedan viewed pictures of my heart and stated with complete confidence, "You know you're going to have to replace this valve." Those were the first words he ever spoke to me. Last year I had no symptoms. I was determined to prove him wrong.

This year was different.

Dr. Kedan explained that, in the past year, stenosis, a stiffening and reduction of the valve opening due to calcium deposits, had significantly decreased the flow of blood through my heart. An opening that should be 3 cm square had now shrunk to .7 cm, less than a third of normal size. My condition was now considered critical. I was living in the danger zone.

I told Dr. Kedan about the burning in my chest and my rapid heartbeat on the golf course. He was certain that they were warning signs, symptoms of the condition of the valve. I wanted to tell him he was wrong. But I knew he was right. I really didn't have an option. If I decided to do nothing and forego the surgery, I would probably die from a massive heart attack within three years. Holy shit. I couldn't believe it. I was going to have open-heart surgery.

Dr. Kedan asked if there was a surgeon I had in mind. Just a few years ago, my dear friend, Lois Wellen, had her aortic valve successfully replaced at Cedars-Sinai by Dr. Alfredo Trento. Her husband, Rob, who I've known since the fifth grade in Long Beach, raved about him. Lois is diabetic and struggles with numerous physical ailments.

"If Lois could have a positive outcome from the procedure," Rob stated confidently, "there was no reason you shouldn't." Dr. Kedan thought Dr. Trento was an excellent idea. He'd arrange a consultation.

Two days later, I had an angiogram, a non-invasive procedure to x-ray my heart, at Cedars-Sinai Medical Center in Los Angeles. After a short wait in pre-op, an operating room became available and I was wheeled away. Lying on the gurney, I gazed at the acoustical tiled ceiling and the fluorescent lights overhead. I felt like a day player in an "E.R." episode. Before I knew it, I arrived at my destination.

Dr. Kedan gave me a mild sedative and carefully inserted a catheter into the femoral artery in my groin. He then proceeded to release a dye to visualize my blood vessels and give him the pictures and the information he needed.

I turned my head to the left and looked at the monitor. There, in living color, was my heart – beating wildly away. Dr. Kedan began to describe what we were seeing. The heart itself was solid. All my arteries were good except the artery leading to my valve. It was about eighty percent closed. I had two options: insert a stent, a small mesh tube, to open the artery and increase blood flow or bypass the restricted artery with the graft of a healthy blood vessel. A stent would mean medication for the rest of my life. No meds would be needed with a bypass. Since I was already having the surgery, I decided to do the bypass. I was somewhat relieved. My heart was sound, and I only needed one bypass. Hey, it could have been a lot worse. Dr. Kedan informed my wife, Fran, of the results as I was wheeled into post-op. She joined me shortly thereafter and kept me company until I was released a few hours later.

The following day, I was contacted by Dr. Trento's office at Cedars-Sinai and the appointment was made for the consultation. It was scheduled for Tuesday, February 10th at 2:30 p.m. – Fran's birthday. We'd have to wait almost two weeks...

Chapter Two
The Consultation

The two weeks passed rather quickly. I kept busy and decided to play a round of golf the morning before my afternoon consultation with Dr. Trento. Better to be anxious about a missed putt than to be thinking about open-heart surgery. But, to be honest, since I learned of my condition, even if I seemed to lose myself in some activity, the surgery was always on my mind. It was the first thing I thought of in the morning and the last thing I thought of at night.

Fran and I approached the reception area on the sixth floor at Cedars-Sinai North Tower. We informed the receptionist we had an appointment at 2:30 p.m. with Dr. Trento.

The receptionist said, "You mean, THE Dr. Trento."

We were given directions, passed through the double doors behind the reception desk, turned left, and walked down a long corridor to Dr. Trento's office. After filling out some paperwork in the office lobby, Fran and I sat quietly, anxiously awaiting our meeting. A man of about forty suddenly entered, approached the reception desk, and said he needed documentation allowing him to return to work. He was very personable and, while he waited for his paperwork, struck up a conversation. We learned that Dr. Trento had replaced his mitral valve just two weeks before. We couldn't believe it. The entry to his heart was made through the rib cage – less invasive than opening the chest. After he wished us well and left the office, I turned to Fran and optimistically said,

"Maybe this a sign, honey. Maybe the surgery won't be so bad after all."

Before we met Dr. Trento, a member of his staff, Cristina, conducted a basic interview regarding symptoms, medications, the usual stuff. She was warm and possessed a wonderful sense of humor. She assured me that she would be watching over me during my recovery after surgery. I told her I had played eighteen holes that morning and walked the course – pushing my cart along the way.

"Why take the risk?" she said. "Ride in a golf cart, and you'll be just fine."

The interview was over in fifteen minutes and, shortly thereafter, we met with THE Dr. Trento. Dr. Trento was a gracious man, about six foot two, lean, with closely cropped grey hair. The first thing he said to me was, "You look great." I told him I felt pretty great and that's what made my decision so difficult. He took a moment to review my paperwork and explained in very clear terms why the surgery was imperative. He suddenly rose to his feet and said, "Let me listen to your heart."

His first words after placing the stethoscope on my chest were, "You have a very strong murmur." He then added, "Come with me. Let's take a look at your angiogram." Dr. Trento led us to a computer station and called up my file. In less than thirty seconds we were watching video of my heart in action. He pointed to the screen and indicated the arteries on the left side of my heart were excellent. When he pulled up the video of the right side of my heart, he showed me the hardened artery near my aortic valve and the need for a bypass.

Dr. Trento was encouraged that my cardiovascular system was in good shape and my condition was localized to the aortic valve and the artery nearby. We returned to his office. Dr. Trento presented two options for the replacement aortic valve. We could choose an animal tissue valve, either pig or calf, or a mechanical valve, which was completely man-made. The animal valve required no medication. The downside was that it would only last for fifteen to twenty years. The manmade mechanical valve would never need to be replaced, but required a daily dose of Coumadin, a heart medication which would have to be closely monitored and taken for the rest of my life. Secondly, the mechanical valve made a clicking sound. I knew that would drive me crazy. Dr. Trento recommended the animal valve, and my wife and I agreed. Dr. Trento looked over his schedule. Quite to his surprise, he said he could perform the surgery the following Tuesday. I was somewhat stunned. One week! Wow.

Dr. Trento sensed my anxiety and looked for other options. He found a schedule opening two weeks later, February 26th, a Thursday. However, Dr. Trento wanted me to know he had a commitment out of town that weekend and would be unable to personally monitor my recovery from the operation. Fran and I could see he wasn't comfortable with that idea. I asked him what worked for him. He replied, "Next week would be better." I looked at Fran, turned back to Dr. Trento and said, "Let's do it."

I asked if we could replace my valve by going through the ribs and avoid opening my chest. He shook his head. The aortic valve was in the interior of the heart, and the procedure had to be done in the conventional way.

"Is there any way you can do the bypass without removing an artery from my leg?"

He immediately responded with great authority, "Absolutely. I'll use a mammary artery in your chest. Not a problem."

At least I was batting five hundred.

Dr. Trento wanted to make sure there were no surprises when he performed the surgery. In the next few days, I would need to check the carotid arteries that led to my neck and head and have a scan of my heart. I understood the need to check my carotid arteries, but did I really need another heart procedure? Dr. Trento explained that an angiogram only showed the aortic valve from a certain angle. He needed to be certain that my aorta artery was not enlarged. He recalled the untimely death of the late actor, John Ritter, who was also born with a bicuspid valve. As a result, he developed an enlarged aortic artery that tragically ruptured and took his life.

"What happens if my artery's enlarged?" I asked anxiously.

Dr. Trento simply answered, "I'll replace it."

Fran and I rose to say goodbye and thanked him for his time. He looked at me with compassion and said, "I know this is a big deal for you, but we do this all the time." When we returned home, we called family and friends to let them know the surgery was scheduled for the following week.

After I got off the phone, I needed a moment to get my head together. Everything was happening so fast. Just two weeks ago, I went for a routine checkup to my cardiologist and learned my valve had to be replaced. Two days later, I was in Cedars having an angiogram. And in a week's time, I would be having open-heart surgery.

It was absolutely incredible.

Intellectually, I knew this was a preemptive strike to prevent a major catastrophe and improve the quality of my life for years to come. Emotionally, I was totally freaked out. Why was this happening to me? How the hell was I going to get through this? What if something went wrong during the surgery? I quickly realized that those kind of negative thoughts were completely counterproductive and a waste of energy.

I was on the path, and there was no turning back. Let the chips fall where they may.

That night we celebrated Fran's birthday with our daughter, Jackie, and her husband, Lee, at a really great restaurant near our home. Fran wore my birthday present, a beautiful shawl from India that had a design of peacock feathers – greens and purples. She looked radiant.

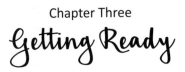Getting Ready

The following morning, I went to see my dentist, Dr. Joel Reims, to check my mouth for any sign of infection. In the event bacteria invaded the heart, it could be life threatening. I've been a patient of Joel Reims for twenty years. He's a consummate dentist and has become a close friend of the family. He's a remarkable guy. He's a passionate sculptor, a special talent that he developed and pursued later in life. I like to think we have an artistic simpatico. I told him that I was about to have open-heart surgery. He asked who was performing the procedure, and I told him Dr. Trento at Cedars.

Joel smiled and simply said he's the best there is. He then asked me what was wrong. I told him I was born with a bicuspid aortic valve that was rapidly deteriorating and had to be replaced.

"Pig valve?"

"I like it better than the mechanical valve. The only bummer is I'll have to replace it again in twenty years."

Joel smiled and said maybe not. He told me his mother had her aortic valve replaced with a pig valve when she was in her late forties. She died at the age of ninety and never needed to replace the valve again. Suddenly, I was feeling better.

I rushed over to Cedars for a bunch of pre-op procedures and then went to the imaging center to have my carotid scan. It was non-invasive, like my echocardiogram. I was concerned about the result and asked the technician if the carotids were okay. He smiled and said, "They're good. Very good." I was feeling much more optimistic. My carotid arteries and the arteries on the left side of my heart were both good. My heart defects were specific, not widespread. I'm going to fix my problem now while I'm healthy and in good shape.

I decided to play a round of golf on Thursday morning with friends Sandy, Mark, and Madison. I rode in the cart with Sandy and felt fine. Sandy Stern has been one of my closest friends for over thirty years. Now in his early seventies, he wrote, produced, and directed countless television movies. He's always writing something and just had his first novel published. The father of four sons, Sandy was a doctor in Toronto before he followed his dream of writing. He had a quadruple bypass over twenty years ago and looks and feels great. He was certain I was going to have a speedy recovery.

After the round, Madison, an actor in his sixties, who's appeared in some of Sandy's movies, joined us for some Zankou chicken on Sepulveda Boulevard. He's a big, handsome guy with silver hair who joins us on the links from time to time. He hits the ball a mile. As we said goodbye, Madison let Sandy know he'd love to play with our foursome whenever there was an opening. I told him that I'd be out of golf commission for about three months. When he learned about my upcoming heart procedure, he shared the fact that he had survived a heart attack. There we were – Sandy who had had a quadruple bypass, Madison who had a heart attack, and yours truly, who was looking at valve replacement and a single bypass.

Madison then cautioned me about the emotional recovery from open-heart surgery. Coming face to face with his own mortality was a very tough thing for him to deal with. I understood. I was already struggling to keep my spirits up and knew it wouldn't be easy.

On Friday the thirteenth, I had an early morning appointment to have a CAT scan of my heart at the Image Center at Cedars-Sinai. This was my last pre-op procedure. I had my fingers crossed that my aorta artery was normal and wouldn't have to be replaced as well.

A dye was injected into my bloodstream that allowed the scan to visualize the heart. A strange kind of warm feeling passed through my body. The tech told me I had a pulse of sixty and my heart was very efficient. More good news.

Later that afternoon, I received a call from Dr. Trento's office. One of his patients needed emergency surgery. My procedure was going to be postponed for one day, and rescheduled for the eighteenth.

I would now wake up from the operation on my sixty-third birthday. A three hundred and sixty-five to one shot came in. Was somebody trying to tell me something? Who the hell knows, but one thing was certain. This would be a birthday I would never forget.

The next day, Saturday, was Valentine's Day. Brother Billy called to invite us to dinner to celebrate my upcoming birthday. Both of his daughters and their husbands were going to join us as well. I was delighted. I told him my surgery had been postponed.

"Can you believe it's the day before my birthday?" I said ironically.

Billy simply replied, "It's the best gift you could ever get."

That Valentine night, the family joyfully honored me at a lovely Italian restaurant in Brentwood and made a toast to my good health. It was just so great to be with everyone. Al Pacino waved goodbye to Billy as he snuck out the door after dinner. Billy leaned over and broke me up with a dead-on impression. His ability to mimic people still amazes me.

The next morning, I continued to do minor errands around the house and garden. I climbed atop the trellis in our backyard and pruned our vines from the side of the garage. Later that afternoon, I whipped up a loaf of no-fat banana bread, which was a lot of fun. That night, Fran and I watched the next episode of "Big Love". It was getting so plot complicated that it became a little too freaky, even for me. As I laid in bed after turning out my night light, I tried to imagine how I was going to handle everything.

And then I thought about my Uncle Berns.

***

For the last twenty years of his life, Bernhardt Crystal spent much of his time in hospitals. He endured numerous stents and other cardiovascular ailments that left him confined to a wheelchair. Towards the end, after his kidneys stopped functioning properly, he dealt with the debilitating effects of dialysis. Even after all those endless procedures, blood transfusions, visits to doctors and specialists, he was still drawing pictures, singing at the top of his voice, or sharing the latest silly joke he had just heard until the very end.

How did he do it?

Of all my relatives, Uncle Berns had the most profound and lasting effect on my life. He was my father's younger brother and worshipped him. When dad tragically passed away, Berns became the patriarch of our family and was deeply treasured as the last Crystal of his generation.

To me, he was "The Great Bernhardt", the heart and soul of New York, my own personal Central Park. He was a larger than life character, much larger than his six foot four frame. He was as strong as an ox and would raise his arms behind his head and make his biceps dance, like they were on a pogo stick. His face was a Mount Rushmore face, bold and filled with enormous character. A Semitic Ernest Hemingway.

In his healthier days, we loved to go for leisurely afternoon strolls in his beloved Gramercy Park. Complete strangers would notice him walking down the street and shout out, "How ya doin' Santa Claus?" Berns would smile approvingly and shout back, "Ho ho ho."

Although he had made his living as an art dealer, he was an artist in the truest sense of the word. He taught me to love and appreciate art, not for its monetary value, but for the way it made me feel when I looked at it. Our home is filled with his art, gifts that he wanted my family to have, works that have enriched our lives. There are tribal masks from Africa in the den, a brass sculpture from Cameroon at the foot of our fireplace, a wood carving from Thailand in our living room, Ernest Fiene charcoals of the East River hanging in the small downstairs hallway, and, my most treasured possession of all, a portrait of me by Joseph Solman that graces our dining room.

When we were young kids growing up in Long Beach, we couldn't wait for Berns to travel from his home in Brooklyn and pay us a visit. We never knew what crazy stunt he was going to pull. He might be dressed in some outrageous costume, make his entrance blowing madly into a slide trombone, or wearing bizarre cardboard masks. He was the original wild and crazy guy, a Marx Brothers movie.

But the ultimate adventure with Uncle Berns was our Sunday trips to visit him on his own turf, his incredible home in Brooklyn. As you might expect, it was filled with amazing art and stunning pieces of furniture. He had this giant circular dining table made of inlaid wood that took your breath away. The centerpiece of his living room was a majestic wraparound couch upholstered in black sharkskin. Behind it were these striking three feet tall Indian sculptures that were positioned dramatically and lit like a museum. He had a lovely garden that ran along the side of his house with a giant white Buddha. It was always a fun place to explore because you never knew what unexpected treasures of art you would find.

His first wife, Ivy, was a bundle of energy and had an infectious laugh. She had this amazing kitchen – professional grade – and was a gourmet cook. When we visited Uncle Berns and Ivy on a Sunday, we never knew what exotic dish she was going to create. It might be an Indian curry, a Caribbean salad with fruits and a variety of nuts, or a raw Japanese fish dish with green mustard and fresh slices of ginger. Each trip to their home in Brooklyn was literally a trip to another world.

Berns loved to perform for anyone who would act as an audience, especially his daughter Dorothy and his adoring three nephews. On those unforgettable visits, we would act out stories and do improvisations. Berns would lift up his voice in song and show me how much fun singing could be. He especially loved traditional spirituals like "I Got Shoes", "Go Tell Aunt Rhody", and "Let My People Go". Although just a young boy with a skinny little body, I could sing in his key and imitate him. He got the biggest kick out of that. He would do magic tricks and use a brown paper bag as a prop. To create the right mood, he would recite an incantation in his deep baritone voice, "Hocus pocus, jiminy ole' smokus, hulabuloo, hulabalai..." and with a snap of his hand, a toy would miraculously appear in the bag. It was an enormous thrill.

Another of his classic routines was the newspaper tree. He would take sheets from the Sunday paper, neatly rolling page after page into a long tube. He would then use his strong hands to tear the top of the rolled up paper in four, equidistant sections. When he was just about ready to sprout the tree, he would ask us to blow into the center of the tube to help it grow. He'd carefully insert his fingers into the torn end of the paper tube and firmly pull out towards the ceiling. We would watch in wonder as the newspaper tree grew to a height as tall as he was.

Years later, when my brother, Joel, and my sister-in-law, Barbara, had children, we would watch with deep affection as Berns grew the tree before their amazed eyes. And when Joel and Barbara's children started their family, Berns performed his trick again. He entertained three generations of Crystals with his magical tree. Like a fine wine, the trick aged timelessly, a treasured family heirloom.

Berns had been a Marine during WWII and witnessed the carnage first hand at Omaha Beach. It changed his soul forever. He became a pacifist, a huge advocate of human rights, and marched on Washington to hear Martin Luther King's "I Have a Dream" speech at the steps of the Lincoln Memorial.

When I was in my early twenties and lived in the lower east side of Manhattan, I would wander up to his stunning gallery on Irving Place and 16th Street. He named it the Washington Irving Gallery in honor of the author, who had lived on the very same block. Berns had this enormous oak coffee table surrounded by black leather chairs where his clients, friends, and artists would spend their weekend afternoons. He'd open a bottle of whiskey, recite ribald poetry, tell corny jokes, and, at the slightest provocation, break into song. No one enjoyed performing for an audience more than my Uncle Berns.

The gallery on Irving Place was extremely successful for many years, despite his lack of business skills. For, first and foremost, my Uncle Berns was a gifted artist. At the age of ninety, he was still creating intricate pen and ink drawings that he would send as a holiday greeting. To Berns, art was as essential to his life as food to eat, water to drink, or air to breathe. Art was his life.

As he neared the end, time chipped away at the handsome mountain of a man and, eventually, reduced him to ashes. He died at the age of ninety-three in his beloved city of New York, one week before our daughter's wedding. Two months later, on the anniversary of his birth, we flew to Manhattan to attend his memorial. Friends and family shared stories about their visits in the gallery, how their homes were filled with his art, and recited off-color jokes. I joyfully led the congregation in song, performing the spirituals he had taught me on Sunday afternoons as a young boy in his home in Brooklyn.

The last Crystal of his generation was sadly gone. My brothers and I had now replaced him as the family elders. I went to sleep that night determined to honor his legacy and make him proud.

***

The week began with a rainy Monday morning. I had an early appointment with my cardiologist, Dr. Kedan. My weight and pressure were excellent. My pulse was seventy-two. Dr. Kedan checked the femoral artery in my groin. It had been three weeks since he performed the angiogram. The entry hole in the artery was healing nicely. My aorta artery was not enlarged and would not have to be replaced. Beautiful. I asked Dr. Kedan if I'd be able to see my aortic valve after they removed it from my body. He said he wasn't sure because it would be taken to pathology. He then asked me if I wanted to hear my heart. He thought it would help me understand why I needed to replace the valve. He handed me the ear plugs and placed his stethoscope on my chest. I heard the eerie sound of a loud breeze that repeated again and again.

WHOOSH... WHOOSH...WHOOSH...

There was no audible beat in my heart. It was very strange.

Dr. Kedan was extremely confident I would have a great recovery. He assured me he'd never have me endure corrective surgery if it wasn't completely necessary. I heard his words and believed they were true. But I still had this tiny speck of doubt. Was I doing the right thing? Did I really need to go through this? I knew it was irrational, but it was a feeling I couldn't control.

On my way out, I noticed a Budget Travel magazine in a cardboard box behind the front reception desk. The word "ITALY" was printed on the cover in bold letters. Before we learned I needed surgery, Fran and I had planned a trip to Italy to celebrate her retirement from teaching the visually impaired for over thirty years. I asked the receptionist if they were throwing the issue out. She smiled and happily gave it to me.

Later that morning, Fran and I drove to Sherman Oaks in the pouring rain to visit Jackie and Lee in their new home. They had recently installed sliding closet doors with opaque glass in their bedroom. It looked fantastic. They also had rented a dumpster bin and had finally removed all the debris from their remodel. The place was really coming together.

Lee showed me an amazing x-ray of a surgery he endured as a young man. Three surgeons worked on him for eight hours to correct a severe curvature of the spine. A metal brace was implanted in his back. Huge screws anchored the brace to his spine and straightened the curve. In order to insert the support properly, they had to collapse a lung and actually move many of his internal organs out of the way. Lee wanted me to know that, if he could survive his ordeal, I would be able to survive mine. It was a lovely gesture. We had a simple lunch at a nearby deli and the rain finally let up.

As the word spread about my condition through our social network, the phone had been continually ringing with concern. Everyone wanted to be notified about the outcome of my surgery. That afternoon, Fran created an email list of friends and family. In this way, she could send a recovery update with one note. It was a great idea. Tuesday would have been a golf day, but the course was wet from the rain. To my surprise, the day went by rather quickly. On the eve of my surgery, Fran and I had a quiet dinner at home and stayed with our usual routine. I turned on the Laker game and tried to make believe this was just like any other night. I knew it wasn't. I got into bed and tried to distract my mind in a book. I had no idea what I was reading. I turned off the light and looked into the darkness. I sighed with resignation.

Tomorrow morning they were going to crack my chest.

Chapter Four
Showtime

Today was the day.

To my surprise, I had gotten a good night's sleep. I awoke at five a.m. and hopped into the shower. As directed, I washed my chest with an iodine sponge to disinfect the area. As I liberally applied the orange liquid, I realized that this was the last shower I would ever take without a scar on my chest. After I dried off, I stood in front of the floor length mirror in our bedroom and took one last look. My chest would never be the same. I decided to snap a digital photo and record the image for posterity.

Every scar on my body tells a story.

The scar that spreads over my right ankle like a spider's web marks the place where a kickstand impaled my leg one hot summer day in Long Beach. My bike slid out on gravel on the corner of Penn Street and Neptune Boulevard as I rode home from a day at the beach. A small scar shaped like a diamond above my right knee marks the spot where a firecracker exploded and opened my leg one sparkling Fourth of July. The Flag Day incident occurred in the empty lot behind our small house on West Park Avenue. The huge scar that wraps halfway around the right side of my lower torso, like a tuxedo cummerbund, recalled the summer in 1964 when I had kidney surgery to repair a mal-rotated ureter tube. Also congenital. Today they do the same surgery without any incision at all. And last but not least, a small scar chiseled into the side of my right eyebrow when I was a precocious six-year-old. It was a rainy afternoon in our first home in Long Beach on West Park Avenue. Looking to release some pent up energy, I did a front flip off the arm of our living room couch. I landed headfirst on a flashlight that was wedged behind two pillows and almost took out my eye. And now, in just two short hours, a new scar, with its own story to tell, would join my elite group of body markings.

I packed an overnight bag with three pairs of pajamas and some old slip-on loafers that I could easily step in and out of. That was about it. I grabbed hold of the bag, took a moment to study the bedroom, shut the light, and closed the door. Fran and I came downstairs and went about our business. Fran walked our spooky Saluki, Aabby. I fed the koi in our pond in the backyard and retrieved the morning paper on the front lawn. The early morning darkness was now turning into a deep, somber gray as the sun began to rise in the eastern sky.

The surgery was scheduled for eight-fifteen, and we needed to check into the hospital at six-thirty. It was twenty minutes to six, and the hospital was only a ten minute drive. We were right on schedule. Fran made her morning coffee and read the main section of the paper. As is my custom, I grabbed the calendar and sports sections. I appreciate the diversion rather than dealing with the murky state of the world. It was Wednesday, and the crossword was still pretty easy for me to handle. I checked the sports section and made note that the Lakers were on the road playing Golden State. Too bad I'd miss the action. Oh well. At least it wasn't the playoffs. We looked at the clock in our kitchen. It was just past six in the morning. Fran polished off her cup of java, and I nailed the crossword. It was ten minutes after six, officially time to go.

Fran decided to take the paper and made sure to bring the book she was reading to pass the time while I was in surgery. She loves to read. I watch sports and listen to jazz. Fran drove, and I sat beside her. The sky was now somewhat brighter but still gray as we cruised along Beverly Boulevard, heading west, the majestic Beverly Center looming in the distance. As we approached the Cedars-Sinai Medical Center, stately and magical like a medicinal Oz, we put the wipers on to sweep away the light rain that sprinkled our windshield. The amber lamps atop the streetlights were warmly shrouded in morning mist.

We drove to the parking entrance at the south tower and checked in at the lobby entrance. Sure enough, my name was on the patient list. This was really happening. A security officer escorted us to the sixth floor reception area. I joined other cardio patients waiting for their names to be called and taken to pre-op. As Fran and I waited patiently for the moment to arrive, I noticed Dr. Trento, briefcase in hand, make his way inside the double doors leading to the surgical area. He could have been a lawyer or business executive entering his office to start another work day.

It was a little after my arrival time of six-thirty when the reality of my situation really kicked in. My mouth got very dry, my stomach was suddenly filled with thousands of butterflies, and a wave of nervous anxiety swept over me. In less than two hours, I would be lying on an operating table, chest cracked open, a team of doctors huddled around me, delicately removing a part of my body that I was born with. My heart would actually be stopped, and I would be attached to a heart and lung machine to keep me alive.

That was not a comforting image to pop into my head at the particular moment. I looked at Fran and reached for her hand. She could sense my anxiety. "You're gonna do great," she said.

Momentarily, an aide approached me in hospital blues and said, "Mr. Crystal, we're ready for you now." He ushered me inside the double doors that, only a week ago, had led me to the consultation with Dr. Trento. We continued down the corridor to pre-op. I was led to a dressing area, instructed to remove all my clothes, and change into a thin blue robe, color coordinated slippers, and hat.

Now I must tell you, even in this dramatic moment before a major surgery, I was still in touch with my vanity. I had no problem with the robe or the slippers, but I took issue with the puffy blue hat. You see, when my dark curly black hair thinned out a number of years ago, I decided not to fight it but be Bruce Willis cool and buzz cut what little hair I had left. Since that time, hats have become a minor passion of mine. To those who know me, well, sort of a trademark. This hat made me feel silly. Completely out of character. I would never be caught dead in this hat. Not literally, of course. Hell, you know what I mean.

I was very uneasy.

Dr. Trento entered pre-op with a big smile, shook my hand, and told me there was nothing to worry about. How about an aneurism? Blood clot? Stroke? Infection? But, before I could engage him in conversation and have him allay my fears, he was off to wardrobe to change into costume and assume the role of surgeon. Without missing a beat, the anesthesiologist introduced himself and asked if I'm allergic to any medications. I told him no. Like a high class drug dealer, he told me he's got the best dope in town – finest quality – and guaranteed me I won't be nauseous during recovery. I'm up with that.

While this was going on, an aide hooked me up to an IV and handed me a sedative to take the edge off. The procession continued. This was one hell of a production. Dr. Trento's nurse, Cristina, as promised in our meeting, appeared with her smiling face. "You're going to do great," she said. I tried to act as confident as she was. "Your wife wants to see you." To my complete surprise, a tidal wave of emotion rose in my gut, and my eyes filled with tears. Cris looked at me sympathetically.

"God, I wasn't expecting to feel like this," I said. "I don't know if I can see her right now."

"You'll be okay," Cristina said reassuringly.

I took a deep breath and tried to compose myself. I nod. I'm okay. Cristina tapped me on the foot and went to get her. And in a moment, I saw Fran's smiling face appear from around the doorway. A sense of calm came over me. We've been through a lot in our thirty years together, and, when it came to hospitals, for the most part, I was the spouse visiting her. Just a few months ago, right after our daughter Jackie's wedding at the end of September, Fran had a procedure to widen a narrowed bile duct, which had led to a painful attack of pancreatitis. We've had enough of hospitals.

She loved the blue hat. I broke into a smile.

Fran moved beside me, took my hand, leaned over the hospital bed, and kissed me. And there was our daughter, Jackie. Her eyes glistening from emerging tears seeing her dad – the coolest dad in the world I might add – dressed in little boy blue for his open-heart surgery. She loved the hat, too. Tell you what, I'd have to reconsider. This silly blue hat is the ultimate ice breaker.

Let's take a picture! Fran reached into her purse and pulled out our pocket digital. Jackie and Fran snuggled up beside me. I held the camera, extended my arm, and pointed the camera at our three smiling faces.

Click. A memory forever.

Cris returned with that warm smile and said it was time. A final kiss goodbye from the precious women in my life, and they left me to take care of business. I felt like I was going to give a concert and perform for my adoring fans, or lead the Long Beach Marines onto the hardwood floor, dish out ten assists, and score twenty against our rival Oceanside.

It's Showtime.

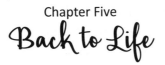

Chapter Five

I felt my body stir, opened my eyes and saw blurry images of light. I closed my eyes briefly then slowly opened them again. A nurse approached me. I looked down and noticed the IV in my arm. I heard voices and the sounds of people moving back and forth as I grew more alert. My surroundings came into focus. In the distance beyond a glass partition, I noticed a team of nurses, doctors, and hospital staff. I was in the critical care unit. My throat was clear. I learned a breathing tube had just been removed. If I was supposed to be in pain, I didn't feel it.

I breathed a sigh of relief. "What time is it?" I asked. It was almost six p.m. There was a drainage tube coming out of my body below my heart that oozed blood into a plastic bag. A catheter had been inserted into my penis to help the drainage from my kidneys.

I felt like Mr. Potato Head.

I tried to get my bearings. Cristina appeared with that ear to ear smile. "Welcome back," she said.

"Everything okay?" I asked.

"You did great!"

I asked for Fran and Jackie and learned that they were with me right after the surgery. I didn't remember that at all. I closed my eyes. The next time I opened them, I was more alert. I noticed a clock in the distance that told me it was after eight p.m. Two hours had passed in the blinking of an eye. I gazed around the room and noticed a television mounted at the top of the wall facing my bed.

Somehow, I had the awareness to remember the Lakers were on the road against Golden State. That meant I could get the game on local television. I pressed the remote on the left side of my hospital bed. In an instant, I was transported outside myself onto the hardwood floor, wearing purple and gold.

How could this be?

Lying with a chest opened on an illuminated table, like some gutted fish, just hours earlier, yet have the presence of mind to remember there's a Lakers game I can watch? Kobe, Pau, L.O., Dfish – No sound. I didn't need to hear the action. Seeing it was enough for me. I tried to keep up with the score, strangely detached from myself and then suddenly realized where I was. What I have been through. The game was too intense. I couldn't keep up with the action. Sorry, Lakers. I had more important matters that demanded my undivided attention.

Click. And the screen goes black.

***

My relationship with basketball began when I was ten years old. I can't remember why or how. All I know is that I fell madly in love. I'd do anything to play. When the school day was over at the nearby East School and it was too cold to play outdoors, I would sneak into the darkened gym through a partially opened side window. Once inside, I'd peek my head into the hallway to make sure Tony the janitor wasn't making his rounds. If I didn't hear the sound of his leather shoes in the distance echoing on the linoleum floor, I'd turn on the lights and begin to practice. I wouldn't dribble or make any other unnecessary noises to give my ruse away. I just shot layup after layup, making sure to catch the ball on its way down before it struck the wood floor. I knew that, if Tony the janitor caught me, I'd definitely be suspended, and my parents would kill me. But that was a chance I was willing to take. For almost three years, I managed to avoid Tony's grasp and never did get suspended. But there sure were a lot of close calls.

There were times in the dead of winter when I actually brought a shovel to the outdoor asphalt court in the nearby schoolyard to remove piles of snow. After a heavy rain, I'd bring a broom to sweep away the remaining puddles, just so I could play. One particular summer, I bought a net that I would attach to the rim on the outdoor court so I could hear the sweet sound of the ball tickle the twine.

I started playing organized ball when I was in the fifth grade, then played on the freshman, junior varsity, and, eventually, varsity teams when I was a student at Long Beach High School. After I was accepted to the University of Bridgeport, I received a partial basketball scholarship from the athletic department. When I took my physical before the start of practice, my doctor discovered blood in my urine. After a series of x-rays, it was determined I had a mal-rotated ureter. The school determined the physical contact of the game greatly increased the chance that I might lose my kidney and made me physically ineligible to be on the team. I was devastated.

Fortunately, my corrective surgery the following June was successful, but my college playing days were over. But, before long, I was back at the schoolyard, enjoying the game more than ever. I continued playing in pick-up games from coast to coast until I was in my late thirties. I reluctantly hung up my high tops when I broke a small bone in my foot after coming down with a rebound and had to wear a cast for six weeks.

It was hard to say goodbye.

Basketball had taught me so many things: discipline, the reward of good preparation, and how to work with teammates to achieve a common goal. It strengthened my spirit and the will to win, which enabled me to do battle in a highly competitive business. But, beyond all of that, it repaid my affection in ways I could never imagine.

After I moved to Hollywood, I quickly realized I needed to do more than just simply wait for the phone to ring for another acting audition. I needed to do something else to make a living. When I told my agent I was going to write, he told me it was the best thing I could possibly do. I decided the best way to jump into this new endeavor was to write what I knew. I knew basketball and had met a lot of unforgettable characters during the many years I had played.

The script was called "Hoops". It told the story of a high school basketball star who missed a last second foul shot that cost his team the championship and how, almost twenty years later, he was still haunted by it. I knew Elliot Gould loved to play basketball and had a lot of heat because of his work in "MASH" and "Bob & Carol & Ted & Alice". I approached Jack Gilardi, an agent at ICM who loved sports, in the hope that he would respond to the material. My hunch was right. Jack really liked it and said he'd get the script to Elliot.

I checked in with Jack from time to time to see if he had gotten a response from Elliot. Not yet. Months went by. I thought the project was dead. Then, I got a phone call from Lou Pitt, one of Jack's colleagues at the agency. They had given the script to O.J. Simpson, who was going to retire from playing professional football with the 49ers and devote all his time to his acting career. O.J. loved the script and wanted to do it with Elliot Gould.

As the weeks rolled by, I kept calling Lou to see if anything was happening with the script. Eventually, I couldn't get Lou to call me back. It was time to move on. It was now pilot season. My agent put me up to be a cast member on a new variety/talk show that was being put together by Westinghouse. It was called: "Everyday". The executive producer, David Salzman, who would later become the television producing partner of Quincy Jones, thought I'd be perfect for the show. He flew me to Philadelphia to do a screen test and see how I fit in with the other finalists being considered to form the company.

The test went well, but they decided to go with Tom Chapin, a talented singer who was the younger brother of Harry Chapin. But, since I had a free trip back to the east coast, I decided to take the train to New York, introduce myself to the New York agents at ICM, and spend some time with the family.

Later that week, I entered ICM's building on West 57th Street in Manhattan to have my meeting. I approached the elevator and the doors parted. I looked up to see O.J. Simpson exiting the elevator, nodding politely as he quickly moved past me. O.J. was in New York to host the Heisman Trophy Awards with, who else, Elliot Gould. I was momentarily stunned. The odds of the two of us being in this particular place at this particular moment had to be divine intervention. I suddenly regained my bearings and shouted out, "O.J."

O.J. turned briefly, waved politely, and headed out the revolving door. I couldn't miss the opportunity and hustled after him.

"Hey, O.J.," I shouted out again. "I'm Richard Crystal. The guy who wrote 'Hoops'."

Suddenly, O.J. stopped dead in his tracks and turned to look at me. His face broke into a warm smile.

"Hey, Richard, how you doin'. I gotta tell ya, man, I really loved your script."

Holy shit, I thought. He really did read it.

"What's going on with that thing?"

"I don't know," I replied. "I thought you could tell me."

"I just left Jack's office. Come with me, and we'll get him off his butt."

Before I knew it, O.J. ushered me into Jack Gilardi's office, and we started talking about my script. I quickly learned Elliot Gould wasn't going to do it.

"I'm sure we can find somebody else," I quickly replied.

Jack looked up for a moment and then turned to me.

"Let me ask you something, Rich. Do you think you could rewrite the script for O.J. to be the main lead?"

"Absolutely," I replied with complete confidence. "In many ways, the story works even better."

I soon learned ICM was setting up O.J. with his own production company and making a huge deal with NBC. It was a great idea. When O.J. and I returned to Los Angeles, we had a series of creative meetings and reworked my story to suit him. O.J. shared stories of guys he played schoolyard ball with as a high school athlete in Oakland that we incorporated into the script. He treated me with great respect and had so much positive enthusiasm for the project that it filled me with confidence.

About a month later, when we locked in the changes to my original screenplay, I found myself sitting in the back seat of a limousine with O.J. Simpson, Jack Gilardi, and Lou Pitt on my way to the NBC offices in Burbank. After some small talk with the executive in charge of movies for television, O.J. went to bat for me. His passion resonated through the room, and, in less than thirty minutes, we had the deal. My first screenplay. My first sale. I was flying high. I did the rewrite in a matter of weeks, and everybody loved it. We planned to start production in a few months. I couldn't wait.

A short time later, I received an unexpected phone call from Lou Pitt telling me there had been a change of plans. O.J. had just read another script called: "Goldie and the Boxer". "Rocky" was a huge hit at the time, and the network and O.J. wanted to seize the moment and felt they should produce that script first. I was disappointed, but they assured me it was just a temporary setback. Months went by. "Goldie and the Boxer" aired on NBC and got terrific ratings. Great news.

Or so I thought.

A short time later, Lou called to tell me that the head of O.J.'s production company had decided that it was in O.J.'s best interests to stay away from sports movies and play other characters. They were afraid he might be typecast. "Hoops" was never produced.

Years later, when I learned of the brutal slaying of O.J.'s wife and Ron Goldman, I refused to believe that O.J. could have done it. He had been so great to me. But then I heard the 911 call from Nicole with O.J. screaming in the background, threatening to break in the door. The complete rage in his voice, the terror it reflected, was a part of his personality that I had never witnessed in all the time we spent together. I was absolutely stunned. I was certain that he did it, and it made me sick to my stomach. The ultimate irony of my bizarre connection to this tragic event is that Ron Goldman's parents, Fred and Patti, were dear friends of my son-in-law Lee's parents, Ellen and Gene Schneller in Scottsdale, Arizona. Fred and Patti Goldman attended my daughter's wedding. Crazy.

O.J. Simpson wasn't the only sports superstar that magically crossed my path because of my love of basketball. The other was Kareem Abdul Jabbar. I first met Kareem in 1965. He was 17 years old, and his name was Lew Alcindor. He was already a legendary basketball player at Power Memorial High School in New York. A close friend and classmate of Billy's, Neil Chusid, had undergone an amazing transition. His family had converted from Judaism to Catholicism. Neil enrolled at Power Memorial High School in Manhattan where he became close friends with "Big Lew".

One particular weekend in early summer, before Lew was to begin his amazing career at UCLA with legendary coach John Wooden, Neil brought Lew out from the heat of the city to the balmy sea breeze of Long Beach.

The whole town was buzzing when they heard that Lew Alcindor was going to play some three-on-three on the outdoor court at Central School. The weekend games at Central School were legendary on Long Island. Great basketball players would travel out from the city in the hot summer months to play some ball and then spend the rest of the afternoon at the beach. On almost every hot Saturday morning, you'd see Al Seiden and Ivan Kovacs from St. Johns, Art Heyman from Duke, and Long Beach's own Larry Brown, then a star at North Carolina, competing to win and stay on the court. It was unbelievable.

And now, Lew Alcindor, the most sought-after high school player in the country, was going to see how he measured up. Whether you were a sports fan or not, to watch this giant swan of an athlete, so graceful, so young, so long, was an unforgettable experience. You knew without a shadow of a doubt that you were watching a future superstar, an opportunity that happened once in a lifetime. Lew spent the weekend in Long Beach with Neil's family and hung out at our house. On Saturday night, there was a party.

Lew was weird and not just because of his unusual size. When I arrived at the party, I found him in dark sunglasses sitting in front of the TV, which had the sound turned off. Thelonious Monk was blaring from the stereo as he watched the action. It was like a scene from an Andy Warhol movie.

I would later learn that Fran had attended the Power Memorial Senior Day at Rye Beach as Neil's date and spent the afternoon with him. I didn't know her at the time, but Fran was at the very same party that Saturday night. Over the years, because of this unforgettable weekend and the fact that Lew was one of Neil's best friends, I felt a connection to his journey and followed it closely. I marveled at his amazing career at UCLA, his confrontations in the N.B.A. with Wilt Chamberlain, Dave Cowens, Nate Thurmond, and Robert Parrish, admired his courageous political views during the Civil Rights movement, and the courage he possessed when he became a Muslim and changed his name to Kareem Abdul Jabbar.

After I moved to Hollywood in 1975, I had the joy of watching his consummate artistry as the center for the Los Angeles Lakers. Somehow, Kareem and I, these two transplanted New Yorkers, had ended up in the same place some three thousand miles from home to pursue our respective careers.

In 1985, our daughter Jackie started kindergarten at the Center for Early Education in West Hollywood. One day she came home from school to tell us that her best friend in class was a young boy named Amir – Amir Abdul Jabbar, Kareem's youngest son. Soon thereafter, at a parent night at the school, Fran and I saw Kareem and reintroduced ourselves. Kareem was still in touch with our mutual friend Neil, who was now living on a kibbutz in Israel. To my complete amazement, he remembered his trip to Long Beach in vivid detail and his brief visit to my family's house on East Park Avenue. He had a fond recollection of my mom and asked me to send her his regards.

A short time later, he invited us to his beautiful home in Bel-Air, and we talked all afternoon – sports, jazz, comedy, politics, the kids, New York, the shows I was producing. It was a wonderful reconnection. Kareem was warm, animated, full of enthusiasm, and possessed an infectious laugh, the complete opposite of his reclusive persona that he was famous for.

In 1988, after Kareem had announced his decision to retire from his basketball career, he called me. The N.B.A. was going to produce a sports video about his life, and he wanted to know if I thought Billy would be interested in doing the narration. I told him I'd look into it. I presented Kareem's offer to Billy, but Billy didn't think it was the right fit. He suggested that it would be great if Kareem told his own story.

I called Kareem to inform him of Billy's decision and his suggestion that it would be great if he could do the narration. It would illuminate the public to the person he really was and would shatter his image of being stand-offish and impersonal. There was a momentary pause as he thought about the idea. Then, he simply said, "I'd like you to produce it."

I was absolutely blown away that he wanted to entrust his life story in my hands, but I doubted I could do it justice. For you see, I had never produced a documentary before. Kareem didn't care. He insisted I was the guy. I knew basketball, loved jazz, grew up at the same time, shit, our kids were best friends. But, most of all, I knew him and made him feel comfortable. I was sold. I laid out the structure for the film, wrote connecting narration, and looked at hours and hours of footage. Not a bad gig for a guy who loved basketball.

When I knew what I needed Kareem to talk about and what footage I needed him to set up, we would get together, and I would shoot in his home, something that no one had ever done before. He was often times moody and hard to pin down, but, eventually, I would get him to focus and talk openly about his feelings. What was it like to be seven feet tall in high school? What was it like to play under the genius of John Wooden at UCLA? What did it feel like to lose your home to a raging fire? To listen to sports commentators criticize you for being withdrawn and too "soft"? I convinced him to talk freely about all these things, and it was a revelation.

After working on the film for a number of months, I rushed to get a rough cut to the production offices at the N.B.A. in Manhattan so we could premiere it at the All Star Game Weekend in Houston. I thought they were going to absolutely love it.

Well, to my shocked surprise, they basically hated it.

As far as they were concerned, the film completely missed. It wasn't hip enough, the jazz score was all wrong, and the piece was much too conventional for contemporary audiences. They were going to fly me to New York as a courtesy and have their editors completely recut the video from frame one. I was stunned to my core. Couldn't eat. Couldn't sleep. I mean, as a producer for hire, you expect to get some suggestions, move a segment here, rewrite here, make this section more clear. Not a problem. I totally got that. But the whole freakin' video? I tried to understand their reasoning. Did they watch the same video that I did? I had poured my heart and soul into this project, and I certainly didn't want to let Kareem down and myself as well.

I decided, for my own peace of mind, to show Kareem the film I had made before it became something else. If he had changes or felt the same way as the suits in New York, so be it. It was his life. We watched the video together in his home, and neither of us said a word. When it was over, he looked at me with a warm smile and simply said, "I love it."

"Well, guess what, big guy. We have a problem."

"Don't worry about it. I'll take care of it."

We didn't change a shot. The film premiered in Houston as promised. The reaction was wonderful. Some months later, "Kareem: Reflections from Inside" won the prestigious International Film and TV Festival of New York Gold Award for Best Sports Video of 1989. It was the highest honor awarded at the festival in the category of sports video. It competed against hundreds of entries from around the world and was scrutinized by panels of judges. For the rest of my life, my experience with Kareem taught me to trust my gut and fight like hell for my creative vision.

Nobody knows anything. They just think they do.

Chapter Six

Rebirth Day

I opened my eyes and things seemed to have slowed down. I looked up at the clock and saw it was ten minutes after twelve. I had been asleep for over three hours. I paused. A smile. It was February 19th. It was my birthday. Happy Birthday to me! I closed my eyes – grateful. Reflective.

I had been in a Sinai hospital before. Mount Sinai Hospital in New York some sixty-three years ago.

***

After a normal birth at Flower Hospital in New York City, I was discharged into my mother's arms and joined the family at our home on Davidson Avenue in the Bronx. When I was one month old, I developed infantile dysentery. A lethal parasite attacked my digestive system, and I quickly became dehydrated. I was admitted to the neonatal unit at Mount Sinai Hospital in critical care. My condition rapidly deteriorated. On April 10, 1946, my father received a Western Union telegram which read:

"RICHARD CRYSTAL IS DANGEROUSLY SICK
COME TO MT SINAI HOSPITAL HOUSE DOCTOR"

Over the next three months, I received fifty-seven transfusions that kept me alive. My maternal grandmother, Susie Gabler, used to call me her fifty-seven kinds. Eventually the medical team at Mount Sinai cured me with mother's milk and saved my life. In June of 1957, when I graduated sixth grade from East School elementary school in Long Beach, Grandma Susie signed my autograph book. She began her inscription by recalling the day she read the telegram and what a blessing my life had been.

At the age of eleven, I didn't fully grasp the meaning of Susie's words. How could I? Grandma Susie was the matriarch of our family. She was larger than life and held court every Sunday at her home that she shared with Julius, my grandfather, her husband of over fifty years. One of twelve children and the mother of six, her house was always filled with members of her adoring extended clan. Although of poor health in her adult years, she'd spend hours in the kitchen preparing mouth-watering meals. No sacrifice was too great for her family.

Grandma Susie was a wonderful storyteller, describing events in great detail, her voice filled with emotion. I used to think that she embellished the severity of my condition to make it more dramatic. I was wrong. After the birth of our daughter, Jackie, my mom gave me the actual telegram addressed to my father from the house doctor at Mount Sinai Hospital. She also gave me a black and white photograph that is now one of my most cherished heirlooms. It's a picture of my mom wrapped in my father's warm embrace at a party celebrating my first birthday. Their smiling faces filled with pure joy.

To think I was loved so much overwhelms me.

In the background, on a table with my birthday cake, stands a toy statue of a lion with a crown on his head – King Richard the Lion-Hearted. It was my Aunt Marcia's idea.

Aunt Marcia was my father's younger sister, with eyes as blue as a clear summer sky that set off her shimmering red hair – a Jewish Maureen O'Hara. She was the devoted daughter of my paternal grandmother, Sophie Crystal.

They lived in adjoining apartments on the first floor at 2270 Ocean Avenue in Brooklyn. On another birthday when I was a wide-eyed boy of ten, my Aunt Marcia took the subway into Manhattan from Brooklyn. She met me at the Commodore Music Shop on 42nd St. and Lexington Avenue, our family business where my father worked as the manager. We walked hand in hand to have lunch at the nearby Hamburger Express. My cheeseburger and fries arrived on a model train that tooted around the counter. After lunch, we took a cab to the Roxy Theatre on Broadway. We saw a live stage show and the movie musical "Carousel" in Cinemascope with Gordon MacRae, a magical memory of my childhood. Although no longer with us, Aunt Marcia would be happy to know it's sixty-three years later and Richard the Lion-Hearted is still carrying on.

***

With my head nestled in a pillow, I heard the faint sounds of life.

Beep. Beep. Beep...

Rustling of people moving quickly back and forth. I sighed deeply. I was okay. I scanned my surroundings. It was ten minutes after five. My head was very clear. I felt no pain. I was surprised I didn't.

A nurse smiled and said, "Good morning, Mr. Crystal. How are you feeling?"

"I think I feel okay."

The nurse pulled my blanket down, emptied the drainage bag, and checked my incision. "Very good," she said.

I had no interest in sneaking a peek at the stitches binding my chest together. Not yet. I shook my head in disbelief. I didn't feel nauseous. I had no dry heaves. Shouldn't I feel like I had to throw up? When I had my kidney surgery in June of 1964, I remembered my body convulsing in violent spasms the days following the procedure. I was certain my stitches would rip open. It was absolutely terrifying. It was due to the anesthesia. But that was forty-five years ago. Why shouldn't I expect that medicine would figure a way to improve the side effects of anesthesia? Hell, if my father was alive today, he would have had a bypass and lived for another twenty years. My kidney surgery kept me in the hospital for almost a month. Today, the same procedure would be non-invasive, and I'd be released in a couple of days max.

Suddenly, the nurse took hold of the blanket and folded it down.

"Time to sit up."

I forged ahead.

The nurse reached firmly behind my shoulder and helped me lift my upper body into a ninety-degree angle. She guided my legs to the left, and they dangled over the side of the bed. I gently pivoted on my butt and looked down at my feet hovering above the floor. Awesome.

"Let's get you on your feet."

"So soon?"

"You'll be fine. How else are you going to sit in this chair?"

I momentarily looked at her like she had lost her mind.

"Give me your arm."

I leaned on her shoulder and gently inched off the bed until my feet touched the floor. I summoned my energy, grunted, leaned forward, and extended my legs. I was on my feet. Shaky. But on my feet. The nurse held my arm, guiding me as I moved cautiously towards the front of the chair beside my bed. She helped turn me around as I bent my knees, surrendered to gravity, and took a seat. I let out a big sigh of relief.

"How you doing?" she asked.

"I'm okay," I said. "Just a little wiped out."

"This will help you build up your stamina."

She handed me a narrow plastic device with three colored balls inside. A breathing tube was attached.

"You need to re-inflate your lungs. This is a triflow spirometer. Breathe in deeply until the first ball lifts into the air."

During open-heart surgery, they stopped my heart to repair it and attached me to a heart and lung machine. My lungs had been collapsed and needed to be inflated again. I was like a car running on tires that were low on air. I took a breath. Nothing. The nurse urged me to try it again. I gathered as much energy as I could and breathed in again. The first ball rose ever so slightly. I breathed out with a sigh of relief and the ball dropped down. I felt exhausted.

"You need to do this every thirty minutes. It's very important."

Suddenly, I coughed. My chest shook violently and I cried out in fear. A little everyday cough that had been a minor tremor had now become a frightening earthquake. My chest felt like it was going to burst apart. She handed me a pillow.

"Hold the pillow against your chest. It will help cushion the shock."

Now she tells me.

"Don't worry. You're not going to come apart. You're doing great."

In an instant, Dr. Trento and Cristina were at my side.

"How's the pain?" he asked.

"I don't have any."

"Very good. Let's remove the catheter and get you eating some food."

In an instant the tube in my bladder was painlessly removed. Hallelujah. Now I could pee in a jar. Dr. Trento moved my hospital gown aside and checked his work.

"Everything looks very good."

"What was the condition of my old valve?"

"Terrible. We should have taken it out three years ago. We'll get you walking this afternoon so we can get you into a room tomorrow. Okay?"

"Whatever you say."

Dr. Trento smiled, tapped me on the foot, and hurried off to surgery. Just another day at the office.

Cristina smiled. "You're doing great."

As she turned to leave to see her next patient, Cristina noted the spirometer and added, "Remember. Every thirty minutes."

I was on my own again, somewhat confused by the speed at which things were moving forward. Didn't I just have open-heart surgery? Within minutes I'm eating yogurt, applesauce, and green Jell-O. Not a problem. I had sat in a chair, could pee in a jar, and had breakfast without any signs of nausea. In a few hours, I was going to be taking a walk. It had not even been twenty-four hours since the end of my surgery. This was crazy. I reached for the spirometer and suddenly remembered that it was my birthday. I should have been taking a breath, making a wish, and blowing out candles on a cake. Instead, I'm watching a colored ball rise in a plastic chamber. Who would have thunk it? And suddenly it hit me that this journey can come to an end at any time.

Sixty-three. How did I get this far? It doesn't seem that old, but, in just twenty years, I'll be eighty-three. And how fast do twenty years fly by? It seems such a cliché Christmas Carol moment – reflecting on my past – thinking about the time I have left. But that's what I was doing. I paused, took a breath, and thought about it some more. What's it all about, Richie? And then I saw my daughter's smiling face. A petite little angel, moving quickly to my side. She looked at me with relief. Beaming. My mind stopped working.

There was only her.

Chapter Seven

Jackie

"Hey, dad," she said. "How's it goin'?"

Her sparkling eyes began to shimmer from tears of joy.

"You look great, dad." She took hold of my hand, leaned over, and kissed me.

"Happy Birthday!"

She had bought me a best-selling mystery thriller – hard cover – and two books of crosswords to help pass the time. It was a quarter after eight, and she had stopped in to see me before her day at her public relations job. It made me feel great.

"How was your night?" she asked.

"I actually watched the Laker game for about two minutes. That was all I could take."

"That's crazy."

"I know. Do you know who won?"

She laughed.

I told her about my morning accomplishments and shared my disbelief at how good I was feeling. She filled me in about the remodel of her new home, her struggles at work, and the antics of her little rescued Yorkie mix, Chloe Lois.

Jackie is everything I want to be.

***

Jaclyn Beth Crystal was born in St. John's Hospital in Santa Monica, California on June 7th, 1980. Fran's labor lasted over twenty hours. We eventually learned it was taking so long because Jackie's little head was stuck in the birth canal. A quick twist of the forceps and out she came. It was exactly two fifty-two in the morning.

The most thrilling moment of my life.

After the birth, as I drove east on Olympic Boulevard to our apartment in Beverly Hills, I was completely overcome with emotion. My adrenalin had been racing for almost twenty-four hours, and I was completely wired. The realization that I had become a dad was frightening. I had no real income. I was an unemployed actor and a writer without a job. How was I going to provide for my family? I was scared to death. I took a deep breath. I tried to stay positive. I reminded myself that I had three feature screenplays under option with major producers. Our lives could change at any moment if I got the call that one of the movies got a green light.

You're going to be fine, Rip.

Fran will be able to take care of Jackie all summer until she returns to her special education teaching position in the fall. At least we'll have her income. Hopefully, something will happen in the next few months. If not, I'll be a stay at home dad. Somehow, someway, I'll figure out a way to make it work. Everything was going to be okay.

It was four in the morning when I got back to our apartment in Beverly Hills. Fran's dad, Joe Agovino, had flown in from Miami Beach earlier that week. Fran was his only child, and this would be his first grandchild. Joe had spent most of the day at the hospital in Santa Monica. But, as the labor dragged on, he grew tired and decided to go back to our apartment and wait for the good news. As I opened the front door, I found him still dressed and lying on the couch. He jumped up to greet me.

"What do we got?" he asked excitedly.

"We got a girl."

His eyes sparkled. He clapped his hands, reached out, and put his arms around me. He was the first person to hear the news. It was great to share this moment with him. Joe and I had a glass of wine to celebrate. We were so excited that there was no way we could go to sleep. It was only five in the morning, but I quickly realized it was eight in New York. I had to call my mom at the house in Long Beach and share the news of this wonderful addition to our family. She was absolutely thrilled that her new granddaughter was named after the love of her life. She couldn't contain herself. This was so much fun.

Being with Joe that night took away all my anxiety. He was a simple man, salt of the earth. He knew I'd been struggling to make a living but always believed in me. He kept telling me to hang in there. I just needed a break.

"Don't worry, Rip. Babies bring good luck."

Joe was one of seven children born to Lucretia and Salvatore Agovino. They immigrated to America from Naples at the turn of the century and settled in Brooklyn. When Joe was a young man, he raised carrier pigeons, baked bread, and loved the Dodgers. He met a Jewish girl in the neighborhood, Belle Miller. They fell in love and remained married for forty-eight years. When he got out of the army, he earned a living as a foreman overseeing the painting of churches in the five boroughs of New York.

He was a fantastic cook. His lobster fra diavolo over a bed of pasta with a tomato sauce made from scratch became a holiday tradition every Christmas. After he retired from the painting business, Joe and Belle sold their home in Long Beach and moved to a lovely apartment near a waterway in Miami Beach. When Fran and I went to visit her parents after they moved to Florida, I asked Joe how he was spending his time.

Joe simply said, "I like to go down to the pier and watch the fish jump out of the water." That was Joe.

Belle had passed away the summer before Jackie was conceived. The prospect of Jackie's birth had lifted our spirits for the past nine months and helped us deal with our loss. It was the perfect antidote to remembering the past. Jackie made us look to the future.

Because of the long delivery the day before, Joe and I were concerned that Fran and the baby were okay. We drove back to the hospital at seven that morning. We hurried to Fran's room, got to the doorway, and anxiously peeked in. Fran was sitting in bed wearing a white nightgown with a look on her face that was unforgettable. She was dreamily gazing down at her daughter, our daughter, tenderly cradling her little pink head in her hands. Jackie was looking up at her mother, completely content, safe, loved, an absolutely magical interaction to behold. Joe and I could not believe how great both of them were doing. The baby was five hours old.

It was a miracle.

Fran went back to work in September, and I took care of Jackie. I had an IBM electric typewriter and worked feverishly to come up with something that would sell. I'd start the day by feeding Jackie a bottle and changing her diaper. Before I would start to write, I would put her in a bouncing seat at my feet as I typed away. It was always a relief when I put her down for her nap and I could work without distraction. Whenever possible, my agent tried to set auditions and pitch meetings after Fran got home at three p.m.

Jackie was such a wonderful addition to our lives, but had also put enormous pressure on me to make something happen. Additionally, our landlord informed us that he wasn't going to renew our lease. House prices were inflating at a rapid pace. We wanted to take the plunge and get into the market. We called my mom and asked if my stepfather, Al Greenfield, would lend us the money needed for the down payment.

Ten years after my dad passed away, my mom was finally ready to share her life with someone new. Two of her three sons had already married, and she was tired of trying to make ends meet. She settled for Al, a distinguished looking Jewish man who made his millions in the garment center. Al offered the prospect of financial security and so she said yes. But she paid a heavy emotional price. Al had never married and had no children of his own. We hoped in time he would become part of our family and embrace us as his own. But he never did.

My mom was in an uncomfortable position. But she wanted to help us and made the request to Al. He reluctantly agreed to lend us the money, but we'd have to pay him back. I assured my mom that was our intention. We knew there were no free rides with Al Greenfield.

A young woman I knew as an assistant at a talent agency was now working as a real estate broker. She began to show us properties. We finally found a cute little two bedroom one bath house in Hollywood. It was only nine hundred square feet, but it had a huge backyard. The previous owner had an assumable fixed loan. This was perfect because I was unemployed. We purchased the home for one hundred thirty-seven thousand dollars and borrowed twenty-three thousand dollars from my stepfather for the down payment. The interest on the loan we assumed was twelve and a half percent. Our monthly mortgage payment was twelve hundred dollars a month.

This would be a huge stretch for us. Our living expenses would more than double. We were scared but seized the opportunity. We had to try to make it work. Besides, we'd be fine as soon as one of my movies got off the ground. We moved into the house in January 1981. Jackie was six months old. My life had changed dramatically. I now had an infant to provide for, a twenty-three thousand dollar loan, and a twelve hundred dollar monthly mortgage payment.

Jackie was a delightful baby. She was beautiful – and had the sweetest temperament. Fran and I were blessed. The months passed by. Our life with Jackie was wonderful. We struggled to make the mortgage payment each month. As the months continued, my projects began to lose their momentum. I did everything I could to keep them alive, but, shockingly, one by one, they all fell apart.

The options on the scripts ran out. Although called back on numerous acting roles, nothing came through. Pressure was beginning to take its toll. My agent told me that a new cable television network, Lifetime, was growing quickly and needed product. Maybe I could come up with something. I decided to create a show about the new world I inhabited as a dad and share the lessons Fran and I had learned. It was called: "What Every Parent Should Know."

Mike Rollens, a television agent at ICM, thought it was a great idea. He knew a producer who would love it and get it off the ground. His name was Woody Fraser. Woody had produced Mike Douglas when he was just twenty-two, helped create "Good Morning, America", and had launched Richard Simmons in syndication. He was known to be a wild man, but a guy who was unstoppable and would get things done. We met at his office at the Gower Studios in Hollywood right before Yom Kippur. He kept me waiting and waiting and waiting. Finally, I got so pissed that I barged into his office. He was sort of surprised – but in a good kind of way. He quickly apologized and just blurted out, "I love the idea. It's terrific. I'm making a deal in a couple of months with Alan Landsburg. When I get over there, we'll put it in development."

What a way to start the Jewish New Year.

As most things in show business, the deal with Alan Landsburg took months longer than Woody expected. But Woody kept his word. He optioned the show, and we began to work together. We had great chemistry. We took it to Lifetime, but it didn't sell. We worked on other projects. I had another idea that Woody loved called: "Nobody's Perfekt". Woody was producing "That's Incredible" at ABC and felt they might be interested. He called me excitedly one afternoon and told me he pitched the idea to the network executives at a run through. They loved it. Woody and I reworked my treatment. The show was now called: "Life's Most Embarrassing Moments."

Certain we had a deal with the network, Woody optioned the show. This was the break I'd been waiting for. Time passed by and no word from ABC about making the show. As weeks turned into months, my elation descended into despair. My confidence quickly disappeared. I couldn't write. I began to see a therapist to try and alleviate my anxiety. I considered going back to school and get a teaching degree.

It was November. Six months had passed since Woody called to tell me that ABC loved my show. We had lived in the house over a year and a half. Jackie was now two. My meager income consisted of some minimal option money and an occasional one day part on a television or movie project. Fran and I were thinking about Thanksgiving, and I wasn't feeling very festive. I had completely given up hope for anything going into production. The phone rang.

"Hello," I said quietly.

"Hey, Rich. It's Woody. We got it."

"Got what?" I replied in confusion.

"Embarrassing Moments. We got the order for a one hour prime time special. We go into production right after the New Year. Congratulations."

I hung up the phone in a stunned silence. Suddenly, the realization began to sink in.

"Holy shit. I've got a job."

This enormous weight that I'd been carrying around for so many years miraculously vanished in an instant. I raised my arms over my head, unleashed a scream of victory and cried tears of joy.

"Life's Most Embarrassing Moments" premiered as an hour special on ABC in the winter of 1983. It was the highest rated variety special of the entire year. It was hosted by John Ritter. The same John Ritter who was born with a bicuspid valve that led to his premature death. The day after the special aired on the network, ABC called to order two more. One of my idols, Steve Allen, was hired to be the host. Over the next three years, I would co-write and eventually produce nine more "Embarrassing Moments" specials.

Within a year, I had paid off the loan to my stepfather. I now had credit, so we could refinance our mortgage as interest rates came down. We started saving money again. It had been seven years since we moved into our little nine hundred square foot home in Hollywood. We began exploring the possibility of moving up to a bigger home. But, any time we found a property we liked, it was out of our price range.

In the summer of 1987, Fran got an unexpected call from her cousin in Miami Beach. Her father had suffered a stroke and was in the hospital. Later that night, Fran took the red eye to Florida to comfort her ailing father. Unfortunately, Joe passed away within a few days. Joe left us a very small inheritance. But, with our savings and the equity in our first home, we were able to afford the house we had always dreamed of: a charming two story structure built in 1927. It has been our home for the past twenty-two years.

Right after we moved in, Fran noticed a white pigeon sitting on the balcony outside our bedroom window on the second floor. For the next few days, the pigeon would coo every morning. And then, as magically as it appeared, it was gone. Never to be seen again. We like to think it was Joe checking in on us and making sure we were okay. I remembered him telling me that babies brought good luck. He was so right. Because Jackie came into my life, I created a show that I never would have thought of before. It took me to Woody Fraser, who launched my career.

***

As I watched my precious daughter walk off to face the world and slay some dragons, I smiled in gratitude for the gift of this young woman in my life. I picked up the triflow and inhaled with all the strength I could summon. The first ball gently rose in the plastic chamber then dropped in an instant. Suddenly, I felt completely drained. I closed my eyes and quickly fell asleep.

Chapter Eight
Heartbeat

A short time later, I opened my eyes and saw Dr. Kedan approaching me. He's an impressive young man, a no bullshit guy with a sense of compassion. I responded to his demeanor from the moment I met him over a year ago.

"So, how's it goin'?"

"Okay, I guess. Quite frankly, I'm surprised I feel as good as I do."

"I told you you'd do great. How are you dealing with the pain?"

"Whatever they're giving me seems to be working."

"Good. You handled the surgery extremely well. So well, in fact, that you didn't need any transfusions."

"That's awesome."

"It's pretty amazing alright."

He leaned over and looked at my chest. The incision looked good and the drainage was working fine. He noticed the triflow beside me.

"Have you started using it?"

"I can get the first ball in the air. But, man, I can't believe how exhausted I feel from taking a deep breath."

"Keep working on it. Before you know it, you'll lift all three."

"I think that's going to take some time."

"You'd be surprised. The human body has a remarkable way of recuperating. It's an incredible thing to witness. Let me listen to your heart."

Dr. Kedan took his stethoscope and placed the silver disc on my chest. He smiled.

"Perfect."

"That good, huh?"

"Remember what it sounded like before?"

"Absolutely."

"Check this out."

Dr. Kedan handed me the ear plugs so I could give a listen.

Ba-boom, ba-boom, ba-boom, ba-boom...

My eyes widened in amazement. I couldn't believe what I was hearing. Buddy Rich was living in my chest. Strong, powerful, right on the beat.

"Oh, my God..." I said loudly.

"Now you know why you needed the surgery." I sat there in awe.

"I'm going out of town this weekend, and I won't be back until Tuesday. My guess is you'll be home by then."

"Really?"

"I think so. Call me if you need anything, but plan on coming to the office the following Monday, okay?"

"Sounds good."

Dr. Kedan walked off to see his next patient. I couldn't get over hearing the powerful sound of my pounding heart. When I heard my heartbeat for the first time in Dr. Kedan's office, just three days ago, I didn't know what a healthy heart should sound like. Now I did. I suddenly understood what the whoosh represented, how sick I really was. The wonders of science had blessed me and granted me years of new life.

Overwhelmed with gratitude, I began to sob. Fran suddenly appeared behind the glass partition that led to my room. Her smile quickly turned to concern as she saw my body shaking and tears streaming down my face.

"Rip, what's wrong?" In between sobs, I tried to speak but couldn't.

"Are you okay?" Fran asked nervously as she grabbed my hand. I nodded yes and tried to compose myself.

"Frannie," I cried. "I have a new heart."

She smiled and breathed a sigh of relief.

"Dr. Kedan let me listen to it on the stethoscope, and it's just so strong, so healthy, so fantastic."

"That's so great, Rip."

We sat there for a long moment without uttering a word. Just holding hands, wiping away an occasional tear. Suddenly, Fran began to laugh.

"You find this funny?"

"I almost forgot," Fran said in surprise.

"What?"

"Happy Birthday!" Still holding my hand, she leaned over and kissed me.

I smiled warmly and simply said, "I love you."

Fran sat by my side as I nodded off for another nap. Every encounter left me exhausted, drained of any energy. I awoke later that afternoon and had a yogurt. My appetite was coming back. The nurse came to see me and decided it was time to take a walk. She showed me how to rotate my body using my left elbow as an anchor and drop my feet over the side of the bed. I extended my arms downward to support my upper body. I summoned up my strength, lifted my butt off the bed, and slid carefully towards the ground. Fran placed my slip-ons under my feet, and I gently stepped into them. I took a breath and rose to stand erect. The nurse firmly gripped the stand that held my IV drip, wheeled it to my side, and issued her marching orders.

"Okay. One step at a time."

I tentatively moved my right foot forward. It wasn't so bad.

"There you go," the nurse added with encouragement.

I moved the left foot. Not a problem.

The nurse led me away from my bed one small step at a time. Everything was stiff and tentative. I was the Tin Man after the rust set in. But, shit, I was walking. We made our way into the main corridor that connected the critical care unit. The nurse continued urging me on.

"Don't be afraid. You'll be fine. I'm sure you've walked before." I turned and smiled sarcastically at her comment. But it was just the distraction I needed. My steps became more relaxed and natural. It was hard to believe that I was on my feet just a day after my chest was cracked open. But, with each small step, I grew more confident and quickly realized I wasn't going to fall apart.

Suddenly, an older man, looking extremely healthy and vigorous, appeared behind me. His cheeks were rosy and his piercing eyes reflected his intense focus and strong will. He was moving quickly using a walker for support. He literally whizzed by. If there was a speed limit in the critical care unit, he was breaking it. The nurse informed us that this determined patient had received a heart transplant just seven days ago. Fran and I watched him lap us again in complete awe. That night, as I laid in bed, exhausted from the day's events, I couldn't help but marvel at the wonders of modern medicine. It seemed like yesterday when Christian Barnard performed the first heart transplant in South Africa. It was four years after my father's fatal heart attack, some forty-two years ago.

***

When my father passed away in October of 1963, my Uncle Milt, my mom's older brother, informed me the family could no longer afford to send me to the University of Bridgeport. I completed my freshman year, then transferred to Brooklyn College as a business major. I was accepted to the School of General Studies, which was basically night school. The tuition was only one hundred and twenty-five dollars a semester, an inexpensive way to get a quality education and not be a burden on the family. The maximum workload was twelve credits. At that rate, it would take me a lot longer than four years to graduate. However, if I maintained a B average for two semesters, I'd be able to matriculate and become a full time student.

In January of 1964, just three months after my father's death, my older brother, Joel, graduated with his degree in art education from the University of Miami. He returned to our home on Long Island and began to look for a teaching position. Fortunately, there was an opening in the Long Beach School system right in town. Joel applied and got the job.

Like most women of her generation, my mom stayed home, raised her three boys, and kept the house together. She wasn't trained to earn a living or pursue a career. Now a widow at the age of forty-eight, mom needed time to emotionally recover from the devastating loss of her husband and figure out a way to support herself. Joel became the breadwinner and gave her that time.

I finished my last semester at Bridgeport in May. A month later, I underwent my corrective kidney surgery in Long Beach Memorial Hospital. I bounced back quickly. After all, I was only eighteen. I managed to spend the rest of the summer working as a cabana boy at the Malibu Beach Club in nearby Lido Beach. That September, I began my new life of living at home and attending night school at Brooklyn College. I enrolled for the maximum twelve credits and attended classes four nights a week.

Since my days were basically free, I began looking for some kind of part-time job to earn some money. Murray Straus, the father of Cheryl, my high school sweetheart, offered me a job at his findings company in the jewelry district of Manhattan. He was a sweet man and accommodated my school schedule with my work hours. It was a way to pick up extra money to cover all my expenses and contribute what little I could. It was the least I could do to help my brother, Joel, who was keeping us afloat with his minimal teacher's salary.

I became a commuter. I rode the Long Island Railroad to Manhattan and worked at Straus Findings in New York during the day. In the late afternoon, I rode the subway to Brooklyn, got off at Newkirk Avenue, and attended my classes at Brooklyn College. After my last class, which usually ended around nine in the evening, I took the subway back to Atlantic Avenue where I would catch the Long Island Railroad train back to Long Beach. This was my routine for the next two years.

It was an exhausting schedule. To save traveling time, I began to spend nights on the living room couch at my Aunt Marcia's apartment on Ocean Avenue in Brooklyn. It was a small one bedroom apartment, and I felt I was an imposition. Fortunately, my Uncle Berns and Aunt Ivy also lived in Brooklyn and had an extra bedroom in their home on East Thirteenth Street and Avenue H. It was actually within walking distance from the campus and was the perfect solution. I maintained a B average and got an Associate Degree in Liberal Arts from the School of General Studies.

In the winter of 1966, I matriculated as a full-time student at Brooklyn College and continued my higher education. The following fall, I took an elective speech course in Oral Interpretation. Students were required to present four different pieces of literature for their classmates during the course of the semester. My professor was Dr. Melvin White, a marvelous, inspirational teacher filled with contagious energy. For my first performance, I chose "The Tar Baby" by Joel Chandler Harris. It showcased my comedic instincts and versatile voice. It greatly impressed Dr. White and delighted my classmates, especially a young woman named Bianca Sauler.

Bianca introduced herself, marveled at the quality of my voice, and asked me if I had ever sung. I told her that I had starred in a high school production of Kurt Weill's "Down in the Valley." Bianca was an opera singer and was set to star in an upcoming production of the Brooklyn College Opera Theatre. She loved my sense of humor and thought I'd be perfect for a part in Puccini's one act comic opera "Gianni Schicchi". With her encouragement, she arranged for me to audition for the director of the company, Karoly Kope. Karoly wasn't concerned that I had never sung opera before. He was looking for a basso with a good sense of humor. Feeling more relaxed, I did an impromptu imitation of Ezio Pinza singing the last sixteen bars of "Some Enchanted Evening." It always made my brothers laugh.

Karoly absolutely loved it. He cast me as Simone, the cantankerous old cousin of Buoso Donati. The production was first rate and played to sold out audiences. Uncle Berns, who was a gifted singer himself, saved the show's program and recently gave it to me before he passed away. On the bottom of the program he wrote in pencil, "Hi, Richard — one of the great experiences of my life — Berns."

Dr. White attended a performance of "Gianni Schicchi" as well. He thought I was extremely talented and suggested I pursue a career in the theatre. He informed me he would be teaching the following summer at the Banff School of Fine Arts in the Canadian Rockies. They had a musical theatre program that was the best he had ever seen. At his recommendation, the Banff School was prepared to offer me a full scholarship that covered all my classes and meals. Dr. White had an extra room in his summer cottage, so I wouldn't have to pay for a place to stay. My only expense would be the Air Canada flight from New York. Dr. White spoke with my mom and told her it was a wonderful opportunity. Not only was everything free, but the classwork was accredited and would be accepted by Brooklyn College. It was like going to summer school in heaven. That sealed the deal.

I purchased my plane ticket with money I had saved while working in the jewelry business. That June, I took flight for the Canadian Rockies. My summer in Banff was the greatest summer of my life. The setting was breathtaking, the environment, completely inspiring. Every morning, five days a week, I had classes in scene study, dance, and vocal coaching. Afternoons were spent rehearsing "Bye, Bye Birdie", the musical theatre production that would tour Canada later that summer. I was cast as Conrad Birdie, the hip-swinging, rock n' roll singing idol. When we performed the show later that summer in Edmonton and Toronto, I received rave reviews from the Canadian press.

I returned to my home in Long Beach and my career at Brooklyn College. No longer interested in pursuing a business degree, I declared my major in Speech and Drama. Full of confidence in my ability as a performer, I asked my Uncle Milt, who was a giant in the music business, how I could audition for shows on Broadway. He told me to pick up a copy of "Backstage" at any street corner newsstand. Audition notices were listed inside. I had never performed in a professional production and was not a member of Actor's Equity. Milt told me to look for open calls where everyone was welcome.

One afternoon, I read a notice in the trades that there was an open call for a Kraft Music Hall television special. They were looking for four young males and four young females to form a singing group not unlike "The New Christy Minstrels." I decided to go.

I quickly learned what I was up against. There were over five hundred singers looking to land the job. I waited for my turn most of the day. Eventually, they called my name. I stepped into the rehearsal studio and met the casting directors and the musical director, Peter Matz. This was the same Peter Matz who had arranged and conducted Barbra Streisand's award winning record albums. I handed my sheet music to the rehearsal pianist and sang "Luck Be a Lady" from "Guys and Dolls." They seemed to really like me. We spoke briefly. I told them that I had spent the summer as Conrad Birdie and was presently a theatre major at Brooklyn College. They asked me to come back the following day.

I sang again and was asked to return again. The original five hundred singers who auditioned had now been reduced to just fifteen finalists. I was among them. On the last day of auditions, I was introduced to the producers, Dwight Hemion and Gary Smith.

After a brief conversation, Dwight and Gary asked me to stand alongside the remaining finalists. I had passed the talent test. Would I pass the image test? They asked if I had an agent. I told them I didn't and was living with my mom on Long Island. They thanked me for my time and said they'd be in touch. I rode the train back to our home in Long Beach and told my family the audition went great. I really thought I might get it.

Days and weeks went by. With every ring of the phone, I became more and more disappointed. Soon the expectation faded away, and I began to accept the fact that I didn't get the job. Weeks later, Billy and I were having a baseball catch on the narrow grassy mall in the middle of Park Avenue outside our house. Suddenly, my mom raced outside the front door. She began wildly shouting out my name, unable to control her excitement. The people from the Kraft Music Hall were on the phone.

Rehearsals began immediately. The original musical special was called: "Give My Regards to Broadway" and featured the music of George M. Cohan. It starred Bobby Darin and Kaye Stevens. We taped the special at the Ed Sullivan Theatre in Times Square. The very same theatre where John, Paul, George, and Ringo had made pop music history just a few years before.

***

I awoke from my magical television memory to find myself resting comfortably in the critical care unit. I looked up at the clock on the wall that was facing me. It was one thirty-five in the early morning. My birthday had come and gone. I was now sixty-three years old. Before I knew it, I would be sixty-four, the title of a Beatles song I first heard that incredible summer in Banff some forty years ago. I shook my head in utter disbelief.

Chapter Nine

Graduation Day

The night was spent in sleep intervals that lasted a couple of hours. The pain was minimal. When I had to pee, I used a plastic bottle and needed no assistance. I was eating, drinking, all in a rather normal routine. This was all better than I had expected. The triflow was on my night table, and I used it as directed. My progress was barely noticeable. It still took a major effort to lift one ball into the air. I wondered if I would ever be able to do two, let alone three. I opened one of Jackie's crossword books and made a feeble attempt to tackle one. My mind couldn't focus.

Dr. Trento and Cristina stopped by early the next morning to see how I was progressing. The incision was clean. No infection. No oozing. I was cleared to leave the critical care unit and move to a regular room. So far, everything was right on schedule. Fran came early that morning and was thrilled to hear the good news. She joyfully shared the many wonderful messages of good will from friends and family. I had a lump in my throat from the outpouring of affection. I'd always been a sucker for sentiment. The best friend Hallmark Greeting Cards ever had. But this emotional reaction even took me by surprise. Friends and family who I always considered dear to me were now priceless.

Fran wanted to know if I happened to watch "The Office" last night. Completely slipped my mind. She commenced to laugh her way through a recap of the episode. I love her laugh. Just after lunch, we learned a room had become available on the sixth floor. Hallelujah!

To commemorate my graduation, a nurse disconnected my IV and set me free. She sat me in a wheelchair and off we went to make the next stop on my road to recovery. The room was on the sixth floor. And, like all the rooms in Cedars, it was private. But even more importantly, it had a window. I could now gaze out at the world and feel part of it again. After I got settled into my new digs, Fran left the hospital to attend to the everyday responsibilities of our home. I could sense her fatigue and told her to take a break. She needed to catch her breath.

I was feeling good. I was a step closer to the real world and was energized by my quick exit from the critical care unit. Until this moment, I had no interest or stamina to talk to anyone on the phone. But now, left alone, I felt the need to speak with one special person in my life. My older brother, Joel, had been anxiously calling every day and speaking with Fran to hear of my progress. He and his wife, Barbara, were in their new winter home in Florida, some three thousand miles away.

***

Joel and Barbara have been married for over forty years and raised two great kids. Their son, Jonathan, recently married, is a successful producer for HBO Sports in New York. Their daughter, Faithe, is the mother of three beautiful children and, like her parents, teaches in the Long Beach school system. Just months before, Joel had an episode and learned that he had cardiovascular disease. He was now on medication and would have to closely monitor his condition. Joel has always been there for me. He drove me to the Kennedy airport and shipped me off to California over thirty years ago.

After Billy and his wife, Janice, moved west less than a year later, Joel was the last remaining Crystal brother to live in Long Beach. He was the son that stayed behind and was there for mom. The son that needed to run an errand, to make repairs, to watch the house when mom spent her winters in Florida. When the tenant in the upstairs apartment had a problem, Joel got the call to solve it. I'm sure there were times when he resented his situation, but he never made Billy and I feel guilty for living so far away.

And that's why I wanted him to hear my voice. To know I was okay. That he was special to me and in my thoughts. My call caught him by complete surprise. I told him my doctors were thrilled with the outcome of the surgery. It was going to take some time, but they expected me to make a complete recovery. I could hear the sigh of relief in his voice. He wasn't getting second hand updates. He was hearing it directly from the source and, indeed, it was true. His kid brother was really okay. I shared my feeble attempt to watch a Lakers game just hours after my surgery. Now he really knew his kid brother was okay. My energy was fading, and I told

Joel I needed to end our brief conversation. He completely understood, thanked me for calling, and wished me well. I hung up the phone and sat quietly by myself. I couldn't get Joel out of my mind.

Joel was the oldest, he was the tallest, and he had been the sickest. He was four years old when I was born and six when Billy came along. He was a talented athlete whose high school career was prematurely ended when he became a victim of mononucleosis – a severe case that left him housebound for two years of his high school career. His energy was low from the constant fever, and he became lethargic and depressed. How awful it had to be to watch his younger brothers free to play outside, compete in sports, go to school dances, movies, the boardwalk... I don't think he ever really recovered from the years he lost – the joy that was suppressed by his insidious infection.

He attended the University of Miami in Florida because his doctors felt he needed a warm climate. He did what he had to do and, eventually, found his calling and pursued his degree in art education. He always had a great hand for drawing. And, for a big guy, he had what we call in sports "soft hands." But, through good times and bad, he always had a great sense of humor. He's the master of a quick quip, a comeback line, witty as a Robert Benchley essay.

When my brothers and I were growing up, we religiously watched Red Skelton, Jack Benny, and Laurel & Hardy. We fell in love with the comedy albums of Bill Cosby, Jonathan Winters, Mike Nichols and Elaine May, Shelly Berman, and Bob Newhart. We memorized every line of the 2000 Year Old Man with Carl Reiner and Mel Brooks, and laughed our way through the history of the United States as presented by Stan Freberg.

One of the routines we made our own was the Nairobi Trio – an ingenuous mime musical piece conceived by the brilliant Ernie Kovacs. It was perfect for us. There were three of us. We came in different sizes. Joel was large, I was sort of medium, and Billy was this cute little bundle of exploding energy. One night, dad surprised us and brought home the record that Kovacs used as the soundtrack to his classic routine – along with three rubber monkey masks. We mastered the routine, found our own little pieces of business, and began performing it at family gatherings at Grandma Susie's. We killed. The laughs were huge and grew and grew as the piece unfolded. The three of us created characters that had distinct personalities and related to each other without a word being spoken.

But my most vivid memories of Joel all relate to his gift: his ability to draw and express himself through his art. In the eighth grade, I decided to run for office in the G.O. (general organization). I was a popular kid and made friends with everyone. My campaign needed a slogan and a poster to promote my candidacy. Joel drew this amazing portrait of my smiling face inside a crystal ball. The copy read, "It's in the future. Crystal for President." I won by a landslide.

When I attended Brooklyn College at night to earn my bachelor's degree, Joel took a painting class towards his masters. He created a dramatic study of Edmund Hall, a great black clarinetist who had played with Louie Armstrong. The oil painting now hangs proudly in my living room.

My most cherished memory occurred in the spring of 1974. Our kid brother, Billy, left a comedy group and decided to go on his own. The group played the college coffee house circuit but hadn't been able to break out. Agents felt that Billy had great potential as a solo performer and advised him to leave the group. It was a difficult decision, but, with a young wife and a one year-old daughter, he didn't have many options.

A short time later, Billy asked me to come to "Catch a Rising Star," a comedy club on the upper east side of Manhattan, to see his debut as a standup. He needed every friendly face he could find to give him a sense of security – although he really didn't need it. He was absolutely brilliant. I knew, as I had known since he hosted the high school variety show in our hometown of Long Beach, that one day my kid brother was going to be a star. It was his destiny. I was so inspired by his performance that I came up with the idea to write a song about a boy born to be a clown.

I decided to call him "Punchinello" – a classic clown persona in Italian Commedia dell'Arte. I basically stayed up all night and finished the song before dawn. It was a magical creative experience for me. I felt it was something special. That very same morning, I raced over to see Joel. I played him the song on my guitar and asked him if he could illustrate the lyrics using Billy as the prototype. How could he say no? I had Joel's illustrations transferred to slides and projected them on a screen when I performed the song in public. Audiences loved it. I thought about recording it, but I wasn't sure. I knew it would be considered non-commercial and a risky investment for a struggling singer to make.

And then, one day, I was sitting at Joel's kitchen table reading Newsday and learned that Toots Thielemans, the world's greatest harmonica player, is performing with his jazz quartet in a small club out on Long Island. Oh, man. The sound of his melodic harmonica playing the theme to "Punchinello" would be a dream come true. To my way of thinking, this was no mere coincidence. It was a sign, an opportunity. I had to go for it.

I knew the odds of Toots playing on the recording were a long shot, but I had to try. If I could get Toots to say yes, I was going to figure out a way to make it happen. That weekend, I drove out to see Toots perform. During a break, I showed him Joel's drawings and asked him if he would play on the session. He loved the idea, was impressed with my passion, and agreed to do it. I couldn't believe it. I immediately contacted my Uncle Milt to help me put a session together and find the right studio to record the song.

I enlisted Tex Arnold, the musical director of "What's a Nice Country like You Doing in a State like This?", to do the arrangement. Billy was now working from time to time as the opening act for Melissa Manchester. I had met members of her band and asked them to do the recording session. They thought it was a great idea and signed on. The final piece to my creative puzzle came completely by chance. I was walking along Broadway near my apartment on West 87th Street in Manhattan and bumped into Leslie Stein, a former classmate from Long Beach High.

Leslie had become a teacher in the Bronx and was leading her young students on a field trip. Her kids were adorable and I had to ask – could they come to the recording studio and sing the chorus with me. Leslie thought it would be great fun. I scheduled the session around lunchtime during the school week so the kids could make it – and make it they did. They had a ball. Uncle Milt ran the session in a recording studio on 57th Street, Toots Thielemans played harmonica, Tex Arnold arranged it, Leslie Stein's kids sang the chorus, and I had my recording. The song was optioned by producer Jerry Weintraub and almost became the basis for an original musical. Unfortunately, it never got off the ground.

Earlier last year, with the technology of the internet, I enlisted the help of one of my former video editors and produced a music video of the recording with Joel's drawings. Last year, I posted the music video on YouTube and surprised Joel at his new home in Florida with a screening of the DVD. It had been over thirty years since he had seen it. We watched our collaboration together. Joel became very emotional and thanked me for bringing our video back to life. A short time later, he called to tell me he screened it for his three grandchildren who were very, very impressed.

***

I looked out at the blue sky outside my hospital room and shook my head. What a lovely day. Fran returned to keep me company later that afternoon. As I informed her that I had spoken to Joel, we were suddenly interrupted by a visitor. He was a young, black man with an enthusiastic smile. He introduced himself as a physical therapist and immediately began leading me in a series of stretching exercises.

Within a few moments, he had me standing on my feet. We began to walk. He assured me I wasn't going to fall apart and led me into the hallway. He observed my hesitant steps and offered words of encouragement.

"Don't make it so tough on yourself. Walk like you always walk."

I took a breath and carried on. My mind was my biggest obstacle. The therapist reminded me not to look down, to keep my head up, and look ahead. I focused all my energy on just that. I could feel the tension leaving my body as I continued down the corridor.

He asked me to pick a destination. "How about the visitor elevators?"

He broke into a big smile. "Let's go for it."

We made it without a hitch. I looked back down the hall and couldn't even see my room. I felt like I had climbed Mount Everest. The therapist asked me if I wanted to rest. Not a chance. I was on a roll and feeling great about it. As we made it to the finish line, I felt relieved and suddenly drained. The adrenaline stopped pumping, and I needed to get off my feet. The therapist saw me safely back to bed and instructed me to walk as often as possible.

"The more you walk, the better you'll feel."

I thanked him for his help and gratefully said goodbye. I never saw him again.

Chapter Ten

"Are You Billy Crystal's Brother?"

Shortly after dinner, Billy and Janice stopped by to see how I was doing. They thought I looked great. Cedars-Sinai has special meaning to my brother and sister-in-law. It's the birthplace of their two grandchildren and their youngest daughter, Lindsay.

Billy noticed the triflow by my bed and asked for a demonstration. He knew I wouldn't want to let my kid brother down. I took the device in my hand, exhaled briefly to release some tension in my upper chest, and relaxed my shoulders. I breathed in with as much energy as I could muster. This time the first ball lifted into the air with a force I hadn't seen before. I now had actual visual evidence that I was getting better. It was a great feeling. Billy, Janice, and Fran shouted words of encouragement. I smiled with renewed confidence and nodded my head. I told them about walking to the elevators earlier in the afternoon and how excited I was about my progress. Billy wanted to see for himself. Not a problem. It was a great walk. As we passed members of the hospital staff, they smiled at Billy in acknowledgment.

After we said goodbye, I told Fran that I wanted to take a different route back to the room. Her husband was definitely becoming himself again. When we returned to the room, I suddenly felt exhausted. Fran leaned over the bed and kissed me goodnight. I told her I loved her and watched her walk into the hallway and disappear from view. Man, was I tired.

The nurse came into my room to administer my medications and made sure I was comfortable. She commented that the staff realized I was Billy Crystal's brother and that she was a big fan.

"Who's older?" she asked.

"I am," I answered proudly.

She emptied the bag that collected the blood that was draining from my chest, put it back in place, and left me alone to get some rest.

***

Having a sibling who has reached extraordinary levels of fame and fortune can have a debilitating effect on your psyche. It's difficult enough to deal with that kind of success in any walk of life, but, in my case, the entertainment business being a business where success is so visible and the fact that I was trying to make my living in the very same profession – well, I must admit, it has not been easy. If we would attend some entertainment function together, oftentimes people would brush me aside to get close to him. You become an obstacle, a distraction, and it makes you feel unimportant.

Billy Crystal's the star. You're not.

Why? I was obviously talented. Managed to make a good living in a highly competitive business. If I eliminated Billy's career from the equation, I would be considered a huge success. What the hell was it?

I remember one Sunday afternoon in Brooklyn, when I was a ten year-old kid, Uncle Berns got me to join him on a duet, and he was laughing as I imitated his big baritone singing voice. Billy, just 8, suddenly began doing impressions, his one-legged tap dance, and making faces. He literally stole the spotlight. I meekly retreated to the sidelines and watched my relatives laugh at Billy's antics. I couldn't compete with his fierce determination. It was a statement that laid the groundwork for the rest of our lives.

Granted, I was talented. I had ambition, and I enjoyed performing. But that's not going to cut it if you're going to compete to be the best. You have to have that drive to be the best, to work harder than everyone else. You can't teach that. It's a part of who you are. It's always been a part of Billy. But what's also been a part of Billy is his exceptional talent. It was always evident.

When I was a senior in Long Beach High School, I was a huge jazz fan. I mean huge. After high school basketball games on Friday nights, I would lie in bed, turn on my clock radio, and listen in wonder to the magical playlist of jazz DJ "Symphony Sid." My classmates were listening to Elvis, learning to play guitar, and sing like "The Kingston Trio." I was practicing riffs on my tenor saxophone and memorizing instrumental solos of jazz greats like Clifford Brown, Stan Getz, Bob Brookmeyer, and Zoot Sims.

But of all the great jazz musicians of that incredible era, Gerry Mulligan was my absolute idol. He had long blonde hair and literally danced with his shining baritone saxophone when he got lost in his melodic improvisations. He was dating the talented actress, Judy Holiday. He was the coolest of the cool. He was so cool that I gave up my lead tenor spot in the high school swing band so that I could play the bari and be like the one and only Jeru. So, when the Daily News sponsored a jazz concert in Madison Square Garden that featured the Dave Brubeck Quartet with guest soloist Gerry Mulligan, I had to go.

To my surprise, the greatest thrill of that memorable night wasn't listening to Gerry Mulligan but discovering an explosive new band led by one of the most exciting trumpet players I have ever heard. His name was Maynard Ferguson. Maynard's piercing high notes broke the sound barrier and lifted the audience out of their seats. It was absolutely amazing. The following morning, I raced to Tilben's Record Store opposite the railroad station in Long Beach and bought a Maynard Ferguson album. I hurried home with the record and couldn't wait to share my discovery with the rest of the family. I played the grooves off that record. Had to hear it constantly. The opening track was a pulsating gospel piece called "Got the Spirit." I was swept away by the driving arrangement and the soaring riffs of Maynard's horn.

Billy heard more than music. To him, "Got the Spirit" wasn't just a series of notes. It was a heated, escalating dispute between a stern, authoritative baseball umpire and a fiery, frustrated batter. As the solos increased their fury, so did the classic argument at home plate. The musical frenzy culminated with the umpire ejecting the enraged batter from the game. It was inspired. Brilliant. Granted, I heard "Got the Spirit" and recognized the greatness of Maynard Ferguson. But a lot of people could do that. No one else could hear "Got the Spirit" and create a completely original comic interpretation of the music. He did this at the age of 15, just a sophomore in high school. This unique, God-given ability, this comic gift, would propel him to stardom and keep him in orbit for a lifetime. Accepting this fact has finally brought me some long awaited peace of mind. But getting to this place and overcoming my jealousy has been a difficult and frustrating process. For, you see, when we were kids growing up in Long Beach, I was the big brother he idolized. I was the star. I was his hero.

Billy Crystal was Rip Crystal's younger brother.

We shared a room together. We played ball together, laughed together, performed together, and cried together. We went to our first baseball game together at Yankee Stadium and watched in awe, as our idol, Mickey Mantle, slammed a home run off the top facade of the third tier in right field. We went to our first live basketball game together at Oceanside High School and witnessed future N.B.A. coach Larry Brown score forty-five points for Long Beach against his arch rival, future New York Knick, Art Heyman.

But everything changed in 1985, when he appeared as a cast member on "Saturday Night Live". "You look mahvelous" became a pop culture phenomenon, and Billy Crystal was red hot. Within months, he became an international celebrity, and the status quo of our childhood was changed forever.

People who had worked with me on different productions, knew me from high school, or were introduced to me at a party, began calling me to see if I could get Billy to read their script, set up a meeting, or see if I could get him to appear on their television show. It was like I didn't exist. I hated it. Still do. The kicker is, if you tell them the truth and really can't help them, they think you're an asshole. If I presented my driver's license or a credit card, or my name came up in an introduction, people would invariably ask me "Are you Billy Crystal's brother?" Sometimes, I would move on with the conversation and never answer the question. Frequently, when I would answer yes, people would shake their head in disbelief. People are really funny when it comes to celebrities.

On one memorable morning, I had just seen a medical specialist in Beverly Hills and went to reception to pay for the appointment. The assistant, an elderly woman, asked for my credit card and began to process the payment. As she waited for the payment to be approved, she looked up at me and said, "You remind me of someone. He's in the movies. Billy... Billy...oh, what's his name?" I had been in this situation countless times before and chose to let her solve the mystery on her own. As she became increasingly frustrated trying to remember Billy's name, I reluctantly decided to help her out. Just as I was about to put her out of her misery, she blurted out, "Billy Bob Thornton!" I erupted in spontaneous laughter.

Somewhat puzzled, she asked why I was so amused. I told her that I was completely surprised by her comparison. In fact, I was the brother of Billy Crystal. It happens quite frequently when people see my name on my credit card. Completely undeterred, the confident woman stated, "You sound like Billy Crystal, but you look like Billy Bob Thornton!"

Sometimes, being the brother of a famous celebrity can be a pain in the ass. Occasionally, it can be the source of unexpected pleasures.

It was Christmas time, 1993, and Billy and Janice invited us to join their family in the Caribbean. We spent two unforgettable weeks on an amazing boat and traveled to the different islands. It was spectacular. Early one evening, after docking the boat in St. Bart's, we decided to get our land legs and venture onto the island. We strolled along the charming, cobblestoned lanes sightseeing, killing some time before our dinner reservations came due at a local bistro. I wandered off on my own, as I am often prone to do, and turned a corner down a dimly lit lane. I discovered an older gentleman in a white linen suit sitting on a stoop.

He was smoking a cigarette, gazing up at a breathtaking rose-colored twilight sky. I immediately recognized this lanky daydreamer as novelist Kurt Vonnegut. One of the reasons I have achieved success as a producer is that I love talented people. So I have no hesitation about introducing myself to people I admire and telling them that I do. I had a great opener with Kurt because a friend and colleague, Bob Weide, had recently produced and directed a documentary about his life that I had just seen and truly loved. Kurt was delighted to meet me and, with a writer's curiosity, asked about my work and what I was doing in this magical isle so far away from Los Angeles.

As we chatted on, I wanted Kurt to know that my brother Billy was a huge fan as well. In fact, we still talked about Ron Leibman's unforgettable performance as Paul Lazzaro in "Slaughterhouse Five". Kurt gazed at my face for a brief moment, immediately saw the family resemblance, and smiled in recognition. He was visibly moved by the adulation and wanted me to know that he greatly admired my brother's work as well. He finished his cigarette and politely ended our exchange. His wife was waiting for him, and he didn't want to irritate her and ruin a perfectly splendid night. I completely understood.

"Send my regards to your brother. I think he's terrific."

67

I was about to say why don't you tell him yourself, but I wasn't completely sure if Billy wanted to be distracted from this precious family time. So not wanting to make any waves, I quickly dashed off. I caught up with the family browsing in a local shop.

"You won't believe this, Billy," I said excitedly. "I just met Kurt Vonnegut."

Billy was intrigued and wanted to hear every last detail. As I was gushing on about this wonderful chance meeting, Kurt casually entered the shop, spotted us in our animated exchange, wandered up behind my brother, and lightly tapped him on the shoulder.

"Excuse me." Billy cautiously turned around and then, seeing this literary icon, broke into a huge smile.

"Hope I'm not interrupting anything, Billy. I'm Kurt Vonnegut. I'm an old friend of your brother's."

Being Billy Crystal's brother has also filled me with enormous pride and given me unforgettable experiences that I could only dream of. The latest of these took place in the fall of 2007. Billy was awarded the Mark Twain prize at the Kennedy Center in Washington D.C. for his contribution to American humor. It was a wonderful honor for our entire family.

The day before the actual event at the Kennedy Center, we had the privilege of a private tour at the Library of Congress. We saw numerous memorabilia of the Commodore Music Shop, including a handwritten note to my Uncle Milt. It was an extraordinary letter written by Billie Holiday, reminding us again that, in 1939, Milt had courageously produced Billie's classic song about lynching in the south, "Strange Fruit."

We were then taken to the sound library where my brothers and I sat in reverent silence as we listened to an original seventy-eight recording produced by my Uncle Milt for the Commodore Jazz Label. We closed our eyes. The recording was so pure you could feel the heat generated by the sounds of the instruments. We were transported back in time to witness these musical giants jamming in the studio. The sweat dripping off their brow, their cheeks puffed out as they blew their horns, their bodies swaying to the pulsating, surging beat of Dixieland jazz.

As if that wasn't thrilling enough, later that night, we attended a special dinner in my brother's honor hosted by Justice Kennedy in the Supreme Court Building. After dinner, Justice Kennedy and his wife invited us into his private office. He was a gracious host and pointed out different memorabilia and began a passionate discussion about one of his loves, baseball.

When the conversation ended, Billy and Janice left with Justice Kennedy and his wife. As we were about to make our exit, I suddenly had this idea that I thought would be worth a few laughs. I quickly sat myself down at Justice Kennedy's desk and picked up the phone, like I was discussing important business that would affect the nation. Joel snapped the photo for posterity. We laughed like precocious kids as we quickly made our exit.

On the last night of this amazing trip, Billy hosted a dinner for immediate friends and family to thank them for their support. We had a couple of drinks, and, finally, Joel and I showed him the photo of me talking on the phone in the office of a Supreme Court Justice.

Billy freaked out. "What are you crazy?" I was surprised that Billy, of all people, didn't fully appreciate the humor in this harmless prank.

"C'mon, Billy, it's funny."

"What if Justice Kennedy walked into the office and saw you sitting at his desk and talking on the phone? What the hell would you say to him?"

In an instant I extended my hand, holding an imaginary phone, and replied, "Justice Kennedy. It's for you."

The dinner table exploded in laughter. Billy completely broke up and all was forgiven. Score one for the Ripper. But I guess that's what I regret most about his fame and notoriety. He lives under the media microscope and no longer enjoys the freedom of anonymity he had before his stardom. He just can't go to a ballgame at Yankee Stadium without the action being constantly interrupted by throngs of fans pleading for him to sign a scorecard or a baseball. I've been at dinners when Billy was approached by thoughtless patrons who couldn't resist the urge to tell him he looked "mahvelous". I've seen the rush of frenzied paparazzi popping their flashes inches from his face. I've witnessed arrogant fans snapping photos on their cellphones as he arrived at airports or went to the local mall to catch a movie.

I marvel at how he keeps his cool. I couldn't do it.

Good or bad, we live in a celebrity obsessed society. He understands that there's a price to pay and lives his life the best way he can. I'm sure

Billy would say that his ability to maintain a stable family life amidst the instability of show business has been his greatest achievement.

Billy married Janice in his early twenties. They have remained together almost forty years and raised two beautiful daughters. Jenny, the oldest, is an actress and now the mother of two adorable little girls. Lindsay, a talented producer and editor, was recently married and due to give birth to her first child in October.

I have been with Billy from the beginning and sat in the very first row as he rose to stardom. And, undeniably, it's been a thrill. At times, I've envied his success, especially when I was struggling to get my career off the ground. But I never felt sorry for myself. I found my own way and managed to build a career.

***

I lay quietly in my hospital bed. It had been a long day. I was completely drained and surrendered to my exhaustion. I closed my eyes and returned to our home on East Park Avenue in Long Beach. It was late at night. Billy and I were lying in bed. We were filled with energy, talking about the events of the day. We couldn't stop laughing. I smiled warmly and drifted off to sleep.

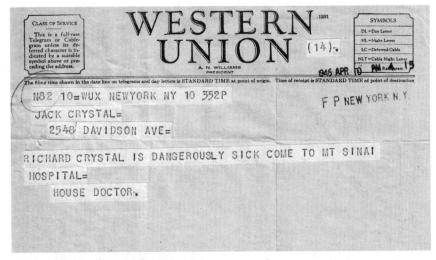

Mt. Sinai Telegram - April, 1946.

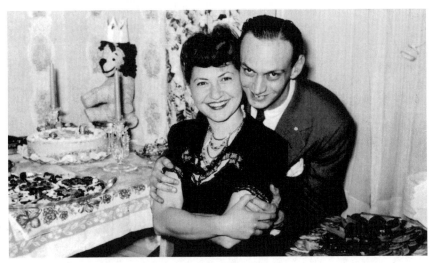

Mom and Dad celebrating my 1st birthday. The toy lion with the paper crown portrayed Richard the Lion Hearted - my Aunt Marcia's idea.

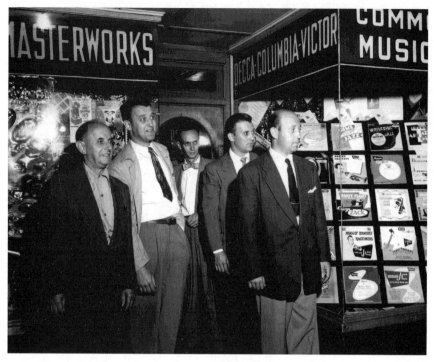

Grandpa Julius with his three sons and dad outside the Commodore Music Shop in it's heyday on East 42nd Street in New York City.

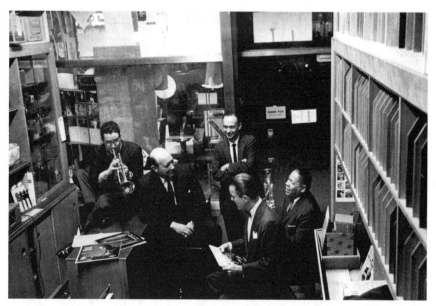

Last Day of the Commodore Music Shop 1958 - Johnny Windhurst with trumpet; Uncle Milt; Dad; Eddie Condon and Henry Red Allen.

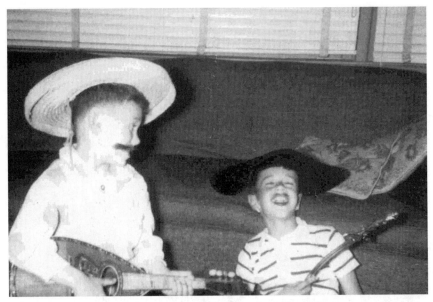
Billy sings Serenade de Muerte as I die from a plastic sword.

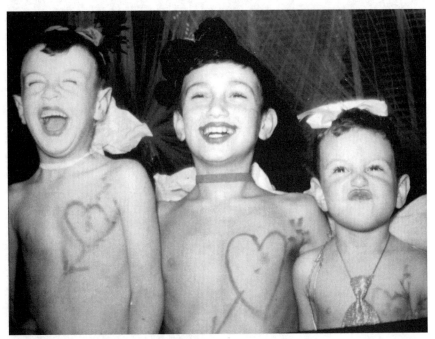
Valentine's Day 1951 - Mom made the costumes and applied the makeup to surprise Dad when he came home from work. Her favorite photo of us as kids.

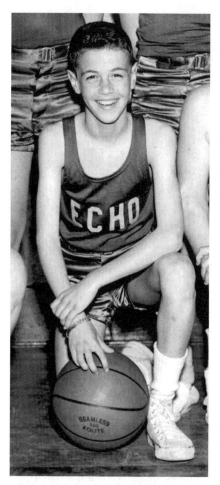

Echo Basketball Team 1959 - my life-long love affair with the game begins.

Shooting a jumper on the court at Long Beach High School.

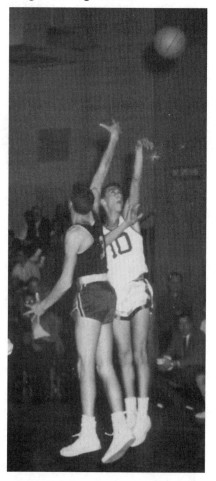

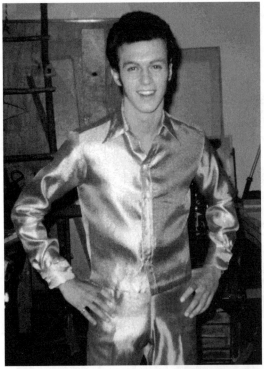

Backstage as Conrad Birdie, Banff School of Fine Arts - Summer 1967.

On the road in Simpsonville, Kentucky singing the Ketchup, Indiana Blues in the Great American Fun Factory - my first Equity job.

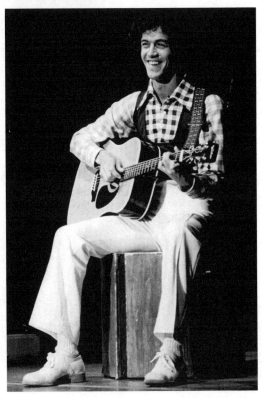

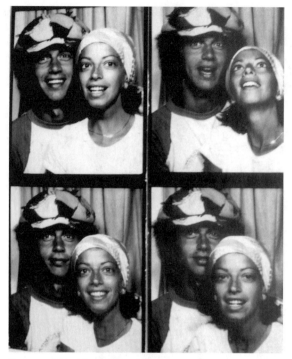

Fran and I in Monterrey, 1975.

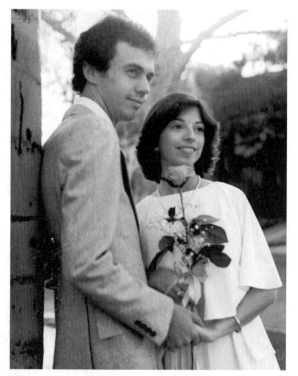

Wedding Day, 1976.

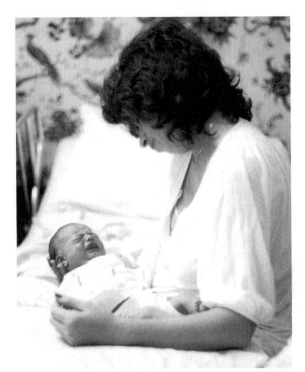

Fran with Jackie, 5 hours old.

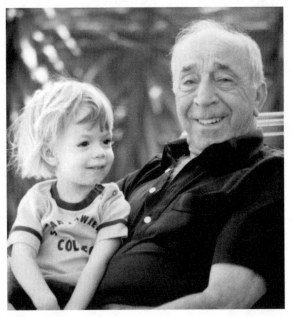

Jackie with Papa Joe.

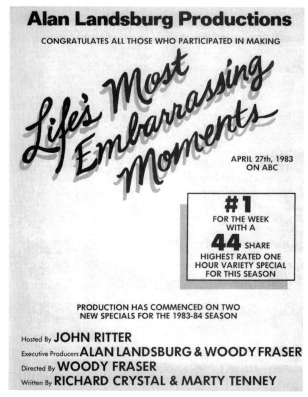

The Big Break, 1983.

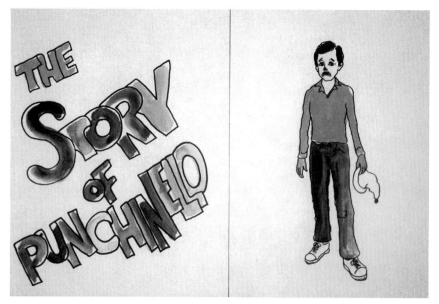

Punchinello - my musical tribute to my kid brother Billy, illustrated by my older brother Joel.

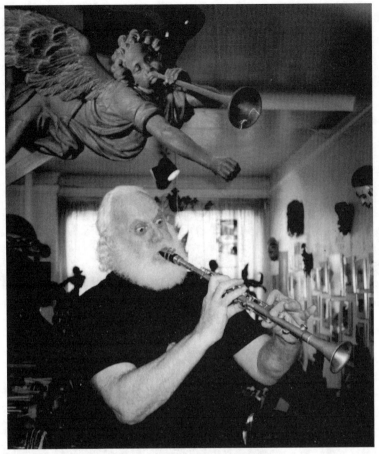

Uncle Berns at Washington Irving Gallery, 1990.

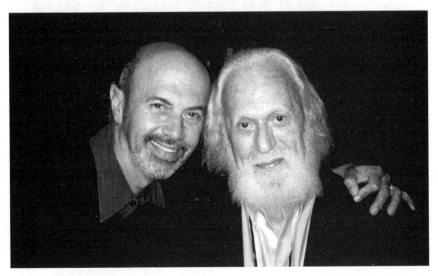

With Uncle Berns on his 90th Birthday.

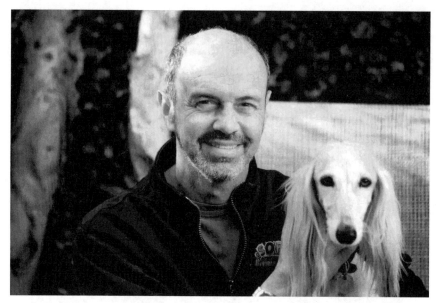

My first Saluki, Aja - Princess of the Desert - named for the Steely Dan album.

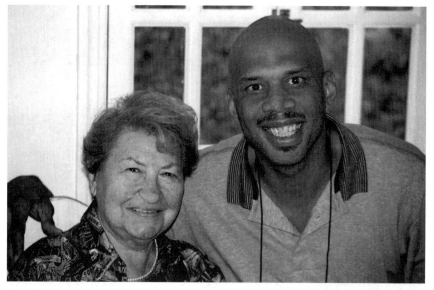

Mom and Kareem, 1996.

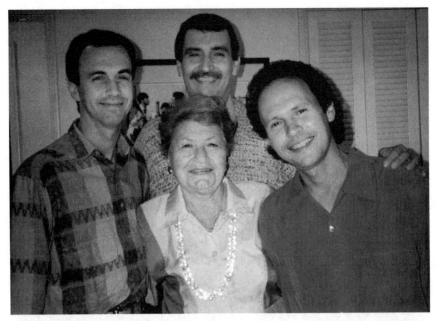

The Big Girl with her boys - Thanksgiving, 1990.

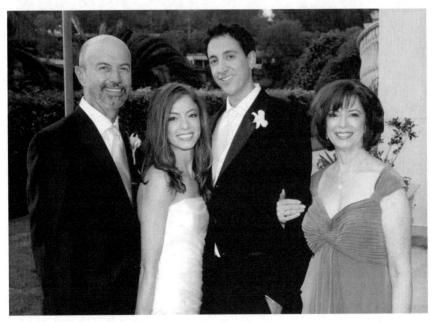

Jackie and Lee's Wedding Day, 2008.

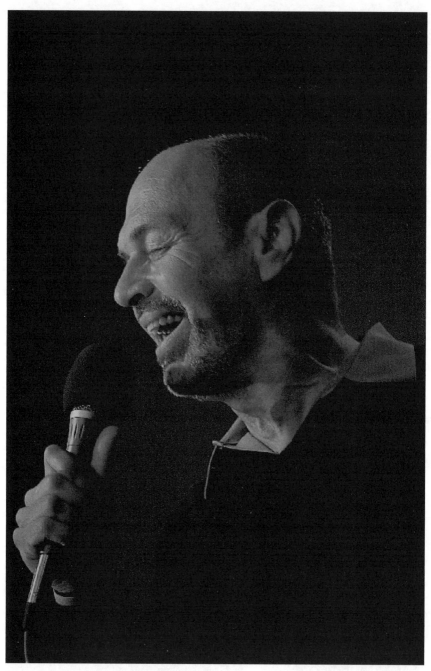

On stage at the Gardenia Supper Club in Hollywood, where Jackie and Lee first met.

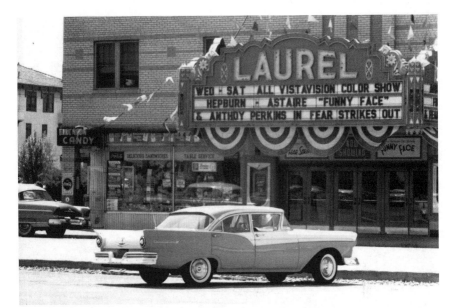

The majestic Laurel Theatre in Long Beach, where I fell in love with movies and graduated high school. Photo courtesy of Dr. K.S. Tydings.

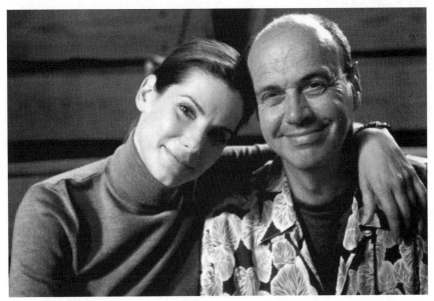

Alongside the wonderful Sandra Bullock on the set of *Murder By Numbers*, which I produced for Warner Bros. in 2002.

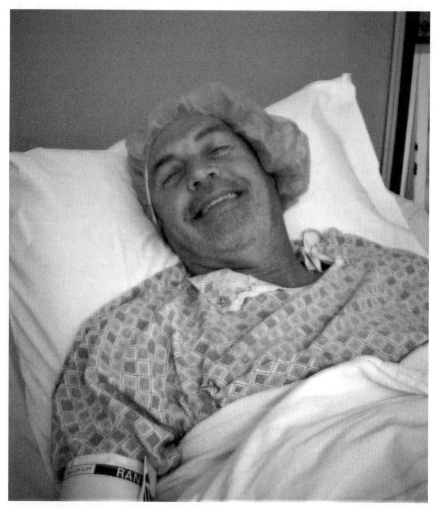

Funny blue hat, minutes before open heart surgery.

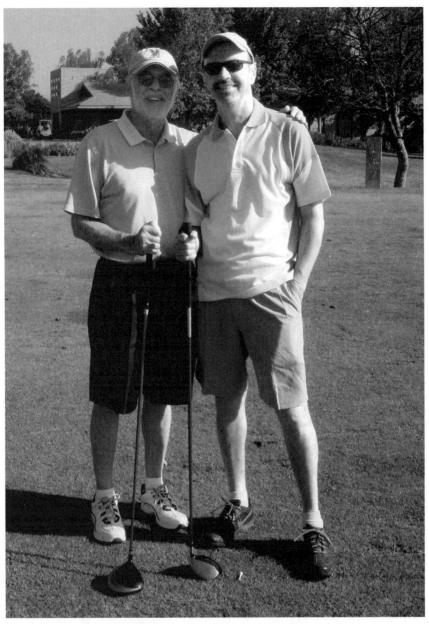
Ready to tee off with Sandy Stern, just three months after surgery.

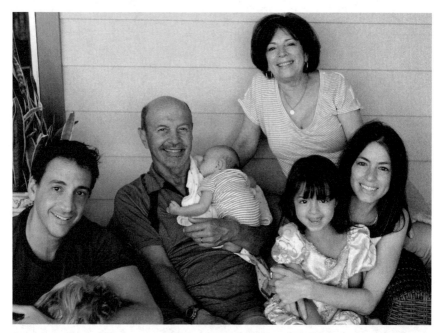

Grandpa Rip holding one month old grandson Maxwell Henry on Father's Day 2015 with Lee, Yorkie rescue Chloe Lois, Fran, Jackie and granddaughter Coco, 4.

Chapter Eleven
A Walk in the Park

Without the constant attention that post-operative patients receive in critical care, Fran was concerned that my first night in a standard hospital room would be extremely rough. We decided to hire a private nurse to spend the night and make sure my needs were promptly taken care of. Her name was Gloria. She was a sweet, middle-aged woman from the Philippines. I would learn that she was wise and had the patience of a saint.

Even though I was on medication to help me sleep, I continued to wake up every two hours. My body temperature seemed to change sporadically as the night wore on, and I'd frequently call on Gloria to wipe my brow with a damp washcloth. After a restless attempt to fall asleep, I found my body uncomfortably twisted at the foot of the bed. Gloria summoned a male night nurse. His name was Julius. He was from the Philippines as well and exuded a knowing confidence and strength.

Together, Gloria and Julius stood by my side, gently reached behind my back, and, with perfect timing, lifted me back to the center of the bed. They were a great team. Julius made certain I was safe and secure, then quickly left to attend to his next medical emergency. Unlike Gloria, this gentle man served an entire floor of needing patients. It was an enormous responsibility, and I marveled at his quiet determination and sense of purpose.

As the night dragged on, Gloria checked the drainage tube in my chest and emptied the bag when necessary. She'd inquire about my needs, encourage me to use the triflow, and made sure my dehydrated body had a continual supply of water. Even though I now had my own bathroom, I wasn't ready to make the midnight run to relieve myself. My sleep medication had transported me into a perpetual state of drowsy. I'd call on Gloria to hand me the plastic urinal that served as my portable toilet.

She sat in a chair at the foot of my bed. When I would grow tired of being awake and nod off, she closed her eyes and stored her energy in a quiet, meditative state. When I awoke at five a.m., I sighed with relief. With Gloria's help, I had safely made it through my first night outside of the critical care unit. She gently administered a much needed sponge bath with a damp wash cloth. It invigorated me and gave me energy. I was ready to start the day.

I called for the triflow. I dug deep to fill my lungs with the air that it so desperately needed. The first ball rose instantly. The second ball trembled and shook from side to side, but never got off its launching pad. I sighed with a brief feeling of exhaustion. Damn, this was tough.

I thanked Gloria for being so attentive and seeing to my needs. She smiled gratefully and said goodbye. It was now time for this caring woman to return home and get some much needed sleep.

The hospital day nurse soon approached me, said good morning, and asked how I made it through the night. She administered my morning medications, took my blood pressure, temperature, and other vital signs. She asked for a fingertip and pricked it with a sharp metal point. A drop of blood quickly appeared and was scanned into a small device to check my blood sugar. I looked down at my fingertips, scarred with black dots. Proof positive that steel pins had pierced my skin and planted numerous flags. My mind flashed back to Victor Mature as a blind, tortured Samson. I saw him being stabbed like a human pin cushion by sadistic dwarfs wielding the sharpened points of lances. A movie moment from my past projected from the recesses of my mind.

The nurse checked my incision. It remained closed and free of any signs of infection. My body was reacting without any serious complications and my pain was under control. The nurse encouraged me to sit in a chair for as much of the day as possible. It would help to increase my stamina and speed my recovery. I slowly swung my legs over the side of the bed, slid down carefully, and stepped into my slip-on loafers.

I extended my arms for support, steadied my legs, and rose slowly to stand erect. I was getting pretty good at this. I looked out at the morning sky, took a deep breath, and stuck out my chiseled chest. I extended my arms and did a series of stretches. I paused to rest. I felt good. I turned away from the window in my room, sighed with determination, and began to walk towards the doorway. Remembering the words of my physical therapist, I put one foot in front of the other, held my head high, and looked straight ahead. I was flying solo.

I said good morning to the nurse at the station outside my room. She applauded my initiative as I moved past her and headed down the corridor. Members of the hospital staff raced by me as I took note of the patients on my floor. It was rather depressing to witness so much pain and suffering. It was just the motivation I need. Grateful to be alive and surviving open-heart surgery was no longer enough. I wanted to get home. I wanted to start the day not by walking down a brightly lit hospital corridor, but on the tree lined streets of our neighborhood with my darling wife, Fran, and our frightfully timid Saluki, Aabby.

***

Aabby is a stunning, tri-color, purebred desert hound with majestic black ears that extend down to the tops of her forelegs. We adopted her when she was three years old to be a companion to our first Saluki, Aja. We got Aja as a puppy. She was a stunning dog, tan like the desert sands. But my loving relationship with dogs actually began many years before.

It had been three years since Jackie was born and we moved into our first home in Hollywood. I now had a production office in Alan Landsburg's building in West Los Angeles and was working on my "Embarrassing Moments" series.

The talented actor, Martin Sheen, had a production company with producer Bill Greenblatt and rented a suite of offices down the hall. One day, Martin's wife entered the building, carrying three little golden puppies in a cardboard box. When I saw these cute little dogs, I melted. The Sheens had already given the pups their shots and were looking to place them in good homes. I called Fran and thought she would love one particular little dog with a patch of white on its chest that had the sweetest disposition.

Jackie was a precious three year old in nursery school. The time seemed right to expand our family. We had an enormous backyard with a giant tree that a dog could call its own. It was a little bit of doggie heaven. Against Fran's better judgment, I brought the little fella home. She knew I made the right decision from the moment she laid eyes on him. Jackie named the golden puppy Sandy because she thought he looked like the dog in "Annie". It was the perfect name. Sandy was amazing with Jackie. She'd yank his bushy tail, but Sandy instinctively knew she never meant to hurt him. He never ever snapped at her. He adored her and always seemed to wear this joyful smile whenever she would playfully tug on his ears. Sandy was a golden retriever/greyhound mix. He looked like a retriever but had a narrow chest cavity. Our backyard was so long that we used to play Frisbee together.

Years went by quickly. Before we knew it, Jackie was in high school and Sandy turned twelve. His energy was suddenly extremely low. He didn't seem to care about exploring or playing as he once did. We were advised to get Sandy a companion and make his life more interesting. Besides, it was the perfect antidote for the guilt we felt when we left him alone. It seemed like a good idea. Fran and I decided to go for it and fulfill my dream.

My mind immediately took me back some fifteen years and recalled a magical moment that I had never forgotten. Jackie was just three months old, and I was walking her in a stroller outside our apartment in Beverly Hills. I suddenly noticed this majestic, regal creature across the street. Its narrow body, proud head, and the delicate grace of its gait took my breath away. I asked the young owner what kind of dog it was. He told me it was a Saluki. I knew from that instant that I had to have one. It was love at first sight. As I wheeled little Jackie back to our apartment, I suddenly remembered that I had heard about Salukis before.

It was 1967. Billy and I went to the N.I.T. College Basketball Tournament in Madison Square Garden. We marveled at the graceful artistry of the amazing point guard of Southern Illinois University, Walt Frazier. The same Walt Frazier who would lead our beloved Knicks to two N.B.A. championships. The Saluki was the team's mascot. But it had no meaning to me then. I returned home and excitedly told Fran of my discovery. I blurted out that if I had ever been a dog in a previous lifetime, I had to be a Saluki. She thought I was crazy and told me that I was smoking too much pot. I was, but that was beside the point. I had never felt this kind of spiritual connection to a dog before. I was intrigued and decided to do some research.

I learned that Salukis were the oldest domesticated breed in the world, their image carved on Egyptian tombs dating back thousands of years. Arab nomads used Salukis to run down gazelles, foxes, and hares in the desert, often with the aid of falcons. Although the Muslim religion considered the dog to be unclean, an exception was made for the Saluki, which was referred to as el hor, the "noble one". Because it helped hunt for food, the Saluki was allowed to sleep in the tent beside its Bedouin master.

Salukis were not allowed to breed with other dogs, which accounted for their purity throughout the centuries. They had no odor, licked themselves clean like cats, and shed very little, if at all. But, if you wanted a dog to fetch a ball, catch a Frisbee, or do tricks, the Saluki was not for you. They're incredibly sensitive, gentle, and have these amazing eyes that look right through you. You get the feeling that they're trying to read your mind or mysteriously trying to understand your inner being. I always thought owning a Saluki was like owning a piece of living art. They are that magnificent.

After waiting almost fifteen years, my dream of owning a Saluki was about to come true. We learned about a local breeder who had some puppies for sale. We excitedly took the drive and brought along our checkbook. The litter was precious. A number of pups appealed to us, but we couldn't make up our mind. The breeder suggested we sit on the floor. The puppy that approached us and overcame its instinctive shyness was the dog we wanted. As soon as we sat down, one little female puppy courageously ventured to greet us. She seemed to love being held and thoroughly enjoyed the affection. I finally had my Saluki. We decided to call the new member of our family Aja. It was the title of one of our favorite Steely Dan albums and was appropriate for her middle-eastern heritage.

From the moment Sandy laid eyes on her, his energy was back in spades. Even though he had been neutered, he tried to mount her every chance he'd get. Fran and I thought he was going to have a heart attack. And who could blame him? Aja was gorgeous, regal, and sweet. A four-legged, mid-eastern princess. Soon Sandy's lust turned to brotherly love. He protected Aja and taught his kid sister what it was like to be a real dog. And, strangely enough, in very short time, Aja became the leader of the pack, and Sandy became one of her royal subjects.

Five years later, Sandy began to deteriorate. He had reached the ripe old age of seventeen. His hips were decaying, and he was in pain. Medication seemed to help, but there were times when I had to carry him into our backyard and physically support him so he could go to the bathroom. Our hearts were breaking, and we decided it was time to put him down. It was hard to say goodbye to our old friend, but we knew it was the right thing to do. No one could have loved a dog more than we loved Sandy.

Sandy's loss had a deep effect on Aja. Although she was only six years of age, she seemed to lose her energy, her youthful playfulness. Every afternoon, she would retreat to Sandy's bed and lie quietly. It was as if she was waiting for him to come home from one of his visits to the vet. We were certain she was lonely and decided to find her a friend.

Aja was so much fun and so easy to take care of that we decided to get another Saluki. The thought of two pieces of art hanging out together in our backyard was wonderful motivation. We knew we didn't want to go through the puppy years again and searched the internet for a Saluki close to Aja's age. We were surprised to learn that none were available. After some time, we discovered a breeder in Orange County that was looking to find a home for a three year old Saluki named Aabby. She had broken her foreleg in her first year. The vet had inserted a steel rod for support, and she was almost as good as new. However, the minor deformity had ended her show career.

Aabby was the last dog born in a litter of nine Saluki pups and the only female. Her brothers were a lot for her to handle, and she became unusually submissive – even for a Saluki. She was one of the most beautiful Salukis we had ever seen, and the breeder assured us that, once the dog got to know us, she would overcome her fears. She never did. But Aabby's submissive personality was just the way Aja liked it.

It was a thrill to watch our two Salukis run off leash in the open desert near Palm Springs – just like they've done for thousands of years. Their majesty, power, and speed took our breath away. About a year after we adopted Aabby and made her part of our family, we noticed a small bump on Aja's snout. Fran and I thought she might have pricked herself on a thorn on one of our rosebushes in the backyard or bruised herself racing through the hard, plastic flap of our doggie door. Thinking the flap on the door caused her injury, we taped it open so the dogs could come in and out with no interference. The bump didn't go away. In fact, it seemed to grow larger.

We took Aja to the vet and, sadly, learned that the bump was actually a mast cell tumor. Unfortunately, it was the most aggressive grade. We considered surgically removing the tumor but decided against it. There were no guarantees she'd be cured and she'd lose an eye. All we could do was treat her condition with medications in the hopes of buying her more time. Eighteen months later, Aja's tumor had grown to the size of a small grapefruit. There was nothing we could do.

With Fran and Jackie at my side, I held my precious Aja in my arms as the vet administered medication to stop her heart. The tears flowed freely as we said goodbye. That was tough. Sandy was almost eighteen when he died. We were lucky to have him as long as we did. Aja's death was much too soon. We had Aja cremated. We planned to scatter her ashes in the open desert where she loved to run free. But we just couldn't do it. Aja's ashes remain in our home to this very day.

***

I reached the elevators and started walking back to my hospital bed. I quickly approached the entrance to my room. An elderly, grey haired woman, accompanied by a nurse, was headed my way. She wore glasses and smiled warmly as we moved towards each other. As we came face to face, I sensed her sweetness, her wisdom, her beauty. Her warm face was etched with wrinkles – each deep, chiseled line telling a story, if you'd take the time to read them. We smiled knowingly as we passed each other in the hall. She was my mother. I was her son.

As I ambled past the nurse's station and entered my room, I felt a sense of accomplishment. And then, suddenly, in an amazing instant, my energy completely disappeared. I couldn't believe it. I was completely wiped out. I paused briefly to catch my breath. What the hell was going on? Hoping to recharge my batteries, I gazed out the window at the blue sky over the buildings on Beverly Boulevard. It didn't seem to help.

I continued on with cautious steps towards the chair just a few feet away. It seemed like forever, but I finally reached my destination. I turned ever so slowly and sank my tired body down into my cushioned oasis. Up until that moment, my recovery was just humming along. I was doing so well. My body had just slapped me back to reality. It was like an army drill sergeant screaming in my face.

"Hey, macho man. What the hell are you trying to prove? You just had your chest cracked open. Remember?"

Yeah, I remember. Thanks for reminding me.

Chapter Twelve

The Big Girl

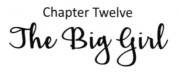

Fran called to ask about my night and if Nurse Gloria had been helpful. I told her I had already taken a morning walk, and she reminded me not to push it. She had to run some errands and would see me in a few hours. I reached for the triflow, took a deep breath, and sucked it up. Still stuck at level one. I felt tired and frustrated. The nurse stopped by to check my pressure, pulse, and blood sugar. This pricking my finger every few hours was getting real old. I was visibly impatient and irritated. Rather than get back into bed and calmly let this gathering storm run its course, I chose to stay in the chair, thinking it would increase my stamina. It was a decision I would later regret.

A dietician soon appeared and ran down my food options for lunch and dinner. Nothing on the menu stimulated my taste buds but, hell, I knew it wasn't Spago. I suddenly remembered sitting with Mom in Long Beach Memorial Hospital a few days after she had her stroke. It was hard to believe it had been over seven years ago.

***

Mom was studying a hospital menu, not unlike mine, with a pencil in her hand. She kept staring at the menu, frozen like a statue, lost in space. Concerned her indecision was a result of the stroke, I calmly asked, "Mom, do you need any help?" She looked up from the menu with a sourful expression.

She simply said, "Would you eat this food?"

I smiled reflectively. A simple question that captured the essence of my mother's spirit. I first learned of Mom's stroke when Joel phoned from Long Beach. Molly Consor, an old friend of Mom's, had anxiously called him when Mom failed to show for their lunch date. Molly tried to reach Mom at home, but her repeated calls went unanswered. Something wasn't right. Joel and Barbara immediately went to check on Mom and found her in the living room, sleeping in her recliner chair. The television was still on, the sound blaring due to her poor hearing. They tried to wake her, but she didn't respond. Paramedics rushed her to the emergency room at nearby Long Beach Memorial Hospital. It was a stroke. She had lost the use of her left arm and was disoriented.

I was in the final stages of post-production for an Animal Planet special and had a deadline that was rapidly approaching. I called my executive producer, Brad Lachman, and informed him of my situation. He offered his sympathies and supported me in any decision I would make. Billy was in New York to see the Yankees play the Diamondbacks in the World Series at Yankee Stadium. It was shortly after the 9/11 tragedy and the city had rallied back to life around the team. He got the call on the way to the game, turned the car around, and raced out to Long Beach. I was torn, feeling terribly guilty I wasn't at my mother's side. But my brothers explained that the doctors were cautiously optimistic. There was a good chance she'd make a full recovery. And, sure enough, Mom defiantly rallied in the next few days. She regained her speech, the use of her arm, and was back on her feet.

I flew to New York at the end of the week to be at Mom's side and fill in for Billy. He had a sold-out concert date in Seattle to perform a show that would later evolve into his award winning "700 Sundays." Joel met me at the airport that Thursday night. I declined his invitation to stay at his home and chose to stay at Mom's. I needed to have my own space and sought refuge in the home I grew up in. He completely understood.

I opened the front door and turned on the light in the foyer. I put my suitcase down on the carpeted floor and stepped into the living room. I stood quietly in a solemn state of reverence and respect. I was standing on hallowed ground. So many years had now passed since I lived there. I breathed in and inhaled the distinctive smells that permeated the musty air like a rare perfume. So unique. So identifiable. I heard the familiar sounds of cars whizzing past the picture window that looked out on East Park Avenue. I was suspended in time, enveloped by the painful awareness that there was one missing ingredient. My Mom.

My eyes immediately focused on the chair in the living room. I saw her sitting there in slumped silence, sucker punched by the sadistic stroke. I was wrapped in a blanket of melancholy. I turned to look at the family photograph on the narrow wall facing her. It's her beloved boys, in the best of times, mugging for the camera on Valentine's Day. Bare chested, hearts drawn with red lipstick and pierced with Cupid's arrows, ribbons in our hair, and angel wings on our backs. A moment of inspired family lunacy. I retreated to the sofa, calmly sat down, and surrendered to my memories.

My Mom was "The Big Girl", the parent who raised us, the mom who had the kids over for homemade cheeseburgers after high school basketball games, the mom that my friends loved to hang out with. She was everybody's mom. She was an exceptional athlete. As a golfer, she had three holes in one. As a swimmer, she won numerous medals. As a bowler, she cracked two hundred countless times, once rolling as high as two thirty five. She taught me how to kick a football on the mall in front of our house. She made us hot chocolate on the cold winter night when we played football in the snow. She came to every performance of every school play. She ran my lines, designed my costumes, and attended just about every game I ever played at Long Beach High School.

And I thought of what a remarkable job she did in raising her three boys. Imagine, her three sons, each successful in their own way. Devoted family men who fell in love with local girls and remained married for over thirty years. Each one raising their own kids and providing them with anything they needed and then some. She was my teacher. She was my nurturer. She was my friend.

I looked at the front door. There was Mom, recently widowed, coming home with a handful of groceries. Suddenly collapsing to the floor, sobbing uncontrollably, overcome with grief that her loving husband was gone forever. I turned my head and looked into the kitchen. The kitchen where she made her cabbage borscht with flanken, franks with beans, and her mouth-watering noodle pudding. Lured by my curiosity, I rose from the couch and walked the short distance to her sacred shrine to get a closer look. The kitchen was so incredibly tiny now. It never seemed that small when I lived there. I noticed the wall phone to my right.

It was suddenly Saturday morning. Sunlight was streaking through the venetian blinds. Mom was sitting on a nearby chair, full of infectious energy, the phone connected to her ear like an umbilical cord, the lifeline to her loving son some three thousand miles away.

"How's it goin', dear? The weather's fine. How's Fran? What's with my little Jackie?"

I looked at the small blackboard on the wall above the kitchen table. A worn out eraser and a broken piece of white chalk rests on the wooden ledge below it. The information desk where we scribbled texted messages, birthday greetings, and thoughtful reminders. Our family cellphone before there were cellphones. My eyes glanced upward to see the familiar wooden paddle of our childhood: "The Board of Education." The board Mom gripped firmly in case of frustration. A loving tool of parental discipline when her boys got out of line. I couldn't help but smile warmly.

I tilted my head down to the kitchen table. I saw mom diligently pounding away on a manual typewriter so she could get a job and keep a roof over our heads. I opened the refrigerator and found her familiar chocolate bar with almonds. I smiled knowingly, broke off a piece, and took a bite. Suddenly, I heard Mom's voice call out to me.

"Rip, dear. Is that you?"

"Yeah, Mom. It's me."

I stepped into the narrow hallway and walked towards Mom's bedroom. My shoulders sagged from the weight of my sadness. I entered, somewhat cautiously, continued to the night table beside her bed and carefully turned on the table lamp. It felt uncomfortably strange, like I was trespassing. What if she found out? I saw her sitting up in bed, her latest book in her lap, anxiously waiting for her son's safe return from another late night out.

I sat at the foot of her bed, like I had done so many nights before, and recalled the heart to heart talks that only we would share. I could always tell Mom anything. I treasured her advice and never felt she wasn't interested or had something better to do. We were very much alike in so many ways. We treated each other with great respect. Our hearts were open books, and we always spoke with complete honesty. We understood each other.

When my teenage heart was broken after Cheryl called from Boston to tell me she had fallen in love with somebody else, Mom was the person I turned to for comfort. When I told her I felt the need to move to California and pursue a career in show business, she didn't tell me don't.

She told me do. When I doubted my talent, she encouraged me. She was far from perfect and wasn't always right. But she was my anchor, taught me how to keep my feet on the ground, and had always been my biggest fan. She was my Mom.

I didn't sleep very much that night. I couldn't wait to see her. The suspense was killing me.

Early the next morning, Joel led me into the critical care unit at Long Beach Memorial Hospital. The very same hospital where my kidney was repaired when I was just eighteen years old. Mom was sitting up in a hospital bed at the far end of the room, her chin resting on her chest. A physical therapist stood beside her, exercising her injured arm. I immediately knew she had been severely damaged. She suddenly raised her head, somehow sensing my presence. Her blank expression seemed to say, "Can you believe it, Rip? I'm so sorry, dear. I don't want to be a burden."

My heart sank. I moved quickly to her side, gently took her hand, and kissed her forehead. She looked deeply into my eyes and just shook her head in a mild gesture of despair. She didn't have to say anything. Fear had shattered her confidence. Although Mom was eighty-five, her mind had kept her young. She was such a sharp woman, so well read, so interested in the world around her. That was no longer enough. I did my best to be strong and conceal my true feelings. She was so frail and disoriented. But what did I expect? The nurse asked for some privacy to change Mom's undergarments, and Joel and I stepped into the hallway.

"You okay?" he asked.

"It's tough to see her like this," I said sadly.

"She's strong, Rip. She's a fighter."

"I know. I guess I had this image in my mind..."

Joel looked over my shoulder and quickly interrupted me.

"Look, at her, Rip. A few days ago she couldn't even stand up. Now she's walking."

I turned around, looked inside the ward, and saw the nurse escorting Mom as she courageously limped forward. A tear came to my eye. She was showing off. Her boys were watching, and she wanted us to know that she wasn't going down without a fight. My worry was replaced with pride.

No one fucks with "The Big Girl".

Now back on her feet, Mom was transferred out of critical care to a general hospital room. Joel and I helped her get settled. It had been an exhausting day. She was worn out and closed her eyes. After dinner with Joel and Barbara, I walked back to the hospital to comfort her. I found her resting quietly. The shock of seeing her condition had thankfully disappeared. I knew what I was dealing with. I studied her face. The paleness that had frightened me earlier in the day had now been replaced by a rosy glow. She remained asleep that night until I left her side. As I stepped outside onto East Bay Drive, there was a spring of optimism in my stride. I made my way back to the house on Park Avenue on a magic carpet of hope.

I called Fran in Los Angeles to share my thoughts about Mom's condition. She encouraged me to be strong, take one day at a time, and let Mom know how much I loved her. I would make the most of this precious opportunity. I got into bed and sat quietly. I was in the small guest bedroom on the west side of the house. It looked vaguely familiar. Not long ago, Billy and Janice had the house completely redone. It was nearing the ripe old age of fifty and needed a facelift. But even though the small space was wearing a different costume, was adorned in the latest style, the soul of the room remained intact. You couldn't fool me. I knew where I was. I knew what it had been.

This was the den, the family room where we watched our small black and white television. I closed my eyes, fastened my seat belt, and traveled back in time. Jackie Robinson's stealing home under Yogi's tag, Don Larsen's pitching his perfect game, Unitas handing the ball off to Alan Ameche and beating the Giants in overtime. I remember laughing at Freddie the Freeloader, loving Lucy, on a second honeymoon with Ralph Kramden, and getting hip with Progress Hornsby. I pay another visit to Ozzie and Harriet, go fishing with Opie in Mayberry, and am reminded that Father Knows Best. It's Friday night once again. Rod Serling spooks me out and Alfred Hitchcock freaks me out. I'm twisting with Chubby Checker, doin' the locomotion, and mashin' potatoes in my penny loafers.

The Beatles are introduced by Ed Sullivan, Jack Ruby appears from nowhere and shoots Lee Harvey Oswald, Neil Armstrong emerges from Apollo 11 to take one small step for man and one giant leap for mankind. I'm suddenly facing Uncle Milt as he solemnly tells me my career at the University of Bridgeport is over. I'm taking a hit on a joint, headset plugged into my Kenwood amplifier. I'm lost in the stoned nasal maze of Bob Dylan, trying to figure out if I'm busy bein' born or busy dyin'. Cheryl lies in my arms after seeing "The Graduate." Just like Benjamin, I've rescued my Elaine.

I crouch down beside my Uncle Berns. This white haired mountain of a man can't bend down and tie his shoelaces. His feet are swollen like two pink water balloons. I opened my eyes and came out of my trance. Amazing. It's still all in there. A DVD in my personal library of life. Saved forever in the hard drive of my mind. I soon drifted away in a deep, restful sleep, embraced by the knowledge that there was no place else I'd rather be.

I awoke on Saturday morning with renewed energy. My emotions were under control, and I was feeling good. Life had thrown me a big fat lemon, and I was determined to make some lemonade. I walked out of the house and headed west on Park Avenue. I turned right on Franklin Boulevard and continued north to the hospital, just a few blocks away. There was a bounce in my step. The sun was shining. A brisk ocean breeze was at my back, and I could smell the salt in the air.

As I walked down the hallway and approached her room, I heard a familiar voice. It sounded just like Mom. No. It couldn't be. I had to be hearing things. Mom was sitting up in bed, talking to her physical therapist. They were planning her rehab schedule, which was to begin later that afternoon. She looked up to see me and welcomed me. "Good morning, Number Two," she said with a warm smile, reminding me that I'm her second born. I had a good feeling Mom was headed in the right direction, but I never expected to see her looking so alert and vibrant.

"I hope my Mom's not giving you a hard time."

"All my patients should be like her."

"How's she doin'?"

"You tell me."

I smile. "She's doin' great."

Mom coasted through the rest of the day. Her instinctive curiosity had magically returned, and she engaged me in conversation, asking about Fran and Jackie, our dogs, my work. Late in the afternoon, she was taking phone calls from concerned relatives. I couldn't believe it. Before I knew it, it was early evening, and it was time to say goodnight. I had to call Fran and share the good news. It was such an amazing day. I had dinner with Joel and Barbara. We were so relieved. Mom still had a long way to go, but she had come so far. Momentum was on her side. We raised our glasses in a toast and clinked them together.

I woke up Sunday morning with a big smile on my face. I took a shower and shaved, looking forward to the events of the day. It was Barbara's birthday. We were going to a matinee of "42nd Street" and then we were going to have dinner in the city. We had some lox, eggs, and onions and then stopped by the hospital to see how Mom was doing. She was sitting up, delighted to see us. Billy had just called from Seattle. His show went great. Completely sold out. Mom wished Barbara a happy birthday and wanted to know about the show we were seeing. Somehow she remembered Ruby Keeler.

But, at times, she seemed confused. She didn't seem as vibrant and alert as the day before. Her quiet demeanor had returned. As we traveled to the city, I voiced my concern. Joel was convinced she was probably just tired from the whole ordeal and needed to catch her second wind. I lost myself in the joy of seeing a Broadway musical and eating a wonderful dinner. It helped me to relax and give my mind a much needed break from my intense concern for Mom. When I returned to the house in Long Beach, I couldn't go to sleep. I picked up the phone and called Billy in L.A.

I shared my concerns about Mom's recovery. Billy always trusted my instincts, especially about Mom, and advised me to speak to her doctors if I sensed she wasn't right. He reminded me that stroke victims have good days and bad days, just like everybody else. He asked me what it was like to stay in the house. I told him I missed the door to our room. He told me I could see it any time I wanted. Unlike my brothers, I was the son who felt the need to have everything around me in its proper place. I was the neat one and loved to make my environment my own.

As kids, we were avid baseball fans and collected baseball cards that we kept in shoe boxes. Not only were the cards great to own and collect, but they also served as the textbooks to courses in Life 101. They taught me the value of something. They taught me how to negotiate. If one of my friends had the card of a ballplayer I wanted and I had the card of a ballplayer he wanted, we'd try to make a deal. Baseball cards also served as my baptism into betting. I gambled on myself, on my ability to stay cool under pressure, as I mastered the art of flipping. Baseball was America's national pastime but flipping for cards was mine. And last but not least, I loved to chew the thin pink slate of bubble gum that came with each and every package. I still have a mouth of silver fillings to prove it. So, to stake out the back room as our personal property, I bought decals of baseball players and applied them to the blonde wood door that sealed our bedroom. It was our signpost. Our "x" that marked the spot. This was our turf. Adults beware. Kids live here.

Years later, when Billy turned fifty, he threw a big bash to celebrate his wonderful life. Mel Brooks took Mom to cloud nine when he asked her to dance. Muhammad Ali appeared unannounced to surprise him and electrify the guests. Robin Williams and Marty Short serenaded him. And his brothers presented him with a gift. The decaled door from the house on East Park Avenue that served as the signpost to our youth. A short time later, he installed it in his home office. It's an emotional anchor. A constant reminder of where he came from.

***

The weekend was over. Monday would be the last day I'd be able to spend with Mom. I had to get back to Los Angeles, put the finishing touches on my Animal Planet special, and deliver it to the network by the end of the week. After we wrapped the production, I planned to return to Long Beach and help Mom in any way I could. When I went to see her early that morning, I grew more concerned. She was clearly more disoriented, more cloudy, more confused. I called her doctor after lunch and shared my concerns. He recommended we do an MRI. It was very likely Mom was experiencing additional mini strokes, like aftershocks of an earthquake. I was relieved he was taking action. His explanation made a lot of sense.

Later that afternoon, Joel and I watched Mom lying on a gurney, being wheeled away to have her brain scanned. There was nothing we could do. We decided to take a dinner break. That night, Joel and I returned to the hospital to see how Mom was doing. She was wrapped in a blanket, bundled up like an infant, looking restful and comfortable. I was happy to see her in this blissful calm. I thought she looked beautiful. She stared at the TV, but I didn't know if she knew what she was watching.

I moved to her side and tried to get her attention. "Mom, how're you doing?"

She didn't respond.

"I won't be seeing you tomorrow, Mom. I have to fly back to L.A."

My words got her attention. She turned and looked at me. She wanted to tell me not to go, but she couldn't. And, maybe if she could, she wouldn't. She turned back to look at the television. Don't ignore me, Mom. I don't want to go. I know you understand. I took her hand and caressed it. I leaned down beside her, kissed her on the cheek, and tearfully whispered, "I love you, Mom."

On the flight back to Los Angeles early the next morning, the image of Mom lying in bed, wrapped snuggly in the bed covers, was fixed in my mind. I lost myself in work that day. It was a good thing. The Animal Planet special was in better shape than I had remembered. I left the office with a sense of accomplishment and relief. We would easily meet our production deadline. I returned home to find Fran cooking dinner in the kitchen. She had been working all day, and it was the first time I saw her since my return from New York. She opened her arms and embraced me. We kissed warmly. We sat down to eat and the phone rang. It was Joel. He struggled to say the words that I knew were coming.

"She's gone, Rip. Mom's gone."

"Oh, no. What happened?"

"She got hit by another stroke. And then another. There was nothing they could do."

Billy called with tears in his voice. He chartered a plane to take us back to New York that night. I would fly coast to coast twice in the same day. It was just the two of us again, sharing a room. There was no way we could sleep. Memories of Mom kept us awake for the entire trip. We laughed, we cried, we shared our sense of loss. Our gratitude. How lucky we had been.

The funeral chapel was overflowing that Friday morning in Rockville Centre. Friends and family traveled from all across the country to pay their last respects. Cantor Richard Botton, who had sung at my Bar Mitzvah and had become a dear friend of the family, conducted the service. Billy took the stage and spoke with warmth and humor, recalling the gifts that Mom had bestowed upon us. Joel shared fond memories of her enduring spirit. Her grandchildren recalled loving memories, and then Billy faced the audience.

"I'd like to call on my brother, Rip. I never saw Mom happier than when she heard him sing."

I climbed the wooden steps to the stage and stood between my brothers for support. I was in the middle where I had spent a lifetime. I looked down at Mom's casket below me, covered in white lilies, and suddenly had trouble breathing. I opened my mouth, but I couldn't make a sound. Tears streamed down my cheeks, and my body shook in convulsive spasms. Marc Shaiman sat patiently at the keyboard, occasionally giving me a brief musical introduction. Billy put his arm around my shoulder and rubbed my back. Joel took my arm and held it firmly. I felt their strength.

"C'mon, Rip. You can do this thing."

I opened my mouth again. I breathed deeply and tried again. I got the first words out, barely above a whisper.

"*You're nearer...*" I sighed briefly and struggled to carry on.

"*Than my head is to the pillow.*" I breathed in again.

"*Nearer. Than the wind is to the willow.*"

And then I found it. The tearful faces of the friends and family looking up at me magically disappeared. I only saw Mom's face. And she was smiling. She was listening to me sing. She was happy. I suddenly felt my body relax. The tears stopped flowing.

"*Dearer than the rain is to the earth below. Precious as the sun to the things that grow...*"

It was just Mom and me. My voice was rich now. I was in control. I knew what I was doing, and why I was doing it. The sound of my soul reverberated through the chapel.

"*Leave us but when you're away, you'll know. You're nearer, cause we love you so...*"

The song had ended. My brothers and I embraced.

Before the casket was placed in the hearse that would take her to her final resting place, we said a last goodbye. Mom looked absolutely beautiful. She was at peace now. Her time had come. Her five grandchildren thanked her for her guidance and wisdom. The three women that had married her sons thanked her for making them feel like daughters. And then, one by one, her three sons bent down and kissed her goodbye.

As a token of our love and gratitude, Billy pulled out a manila envelope, removed a photograph and placed it over her heart. It was the picture of her three boys dressed as cupids on Valentine's Day.

On a cloudy, gray afternoon, Mom was laid to rest at the family plot in the Riverside Cemetery in New Jersey. She joined her parents, Susie and Julius, her brothers Milton, Barney, and Irving, and her sister-in-law, Florrie. But, most importantly, she was buried beside her loving husband, my father, Jack. Finally, after waiting almost forty years, they were together again. It was a wonderful sight to behold.

As we drove back to Long Beach that late autumn afternoon, the dark clouds parted like a gray theatre curtain. A glowing red sun magically appeared center stage and shone brightly in the sky. Heaven was a happier place now. "The Big Girl" had arrived.

Chapter Thirteen

Stormy Weather

I had spent most of Saturday sitting in the chair beside my bed. I had taken a pill for pain right before lunch and was fighting to stay awake. I kept nodding in and out of consciousness like a heroin addict who just shot some bad dope. Fran came to spend the day and brought my iPod. I thought I was ready to listen to music, but that was before my head felt like a bowling ball. For the first time since the surgery, Fran was visibly concerned. She called the nursing service and made sure Gloria could stay with me a second night.

The day nurse looked in on me and directed me to return to bed. When I struggled to get on my feet, my knees buckled. The nurse grabbed hold of my arm and helped me regain my balance. I stopped and took a deep breath. I was frustrated, tired, and grumpy. I got into bed and buried my head into the pillow. Fran approached me anxiously.

"You okay, Rip?"

"I don't know. I feel like shit. I think it's the medication."

A tall, black man wearing a hairnet, gracefully entered my room carrying a plastic tray with my dinner. He's Connie Hawkins long, like a blue heron. He sensed the tension in the room and paused patiently. Fran asked him to place my dinner on the wooden platform that served as my dining table. He gently put it down.

"Enjoy your meal," he added kindly.

He nodded respectfully and retreated quietly. He knew I was in serious trouble. I struggled to eat my dinner. I had lost my appetite. Not a good sign. My temperature was elevated. My body began to ache. I couldn't get comfortable. Fran encouraged me to drink fluids. Maybe I could flush the medication out of my body.

It was almost nine p.m. I had been in this semi-conscious state of pain for almost six hours. The night nurse entered to take my blood sugar. I told her no. Not now. Can't you see what's going on here? The nurse turned to Fran and suggested I take a pill for my pain.

"No!" I shouted out. "No more pain pills! They're killing me!"

Gloria returned at ten p.m. to help me make it through the night. She was surprised to see that my condition had deteriorated. She felt my head and quickly went to get a wet washcloth. I could see Fran was deeply troubled. I asked her to please leave. I didn't want her to see me in my state of distress. She didn't want to go. Gloria assured Fran everything was going to be okay. Fran reluctantly leaned over my writhing body, gently grabbed my hand, and kissed me goodnight. I breathed a sigh of relief when Fran was gone. My body started shaking in painful spasms as tears filled my eyes. I was terribly frightened, stuck in a swamp of quicksand that was taking me under. No matter how hard I tried to claw my way out of it, I kept sinking deeper. My mind tried to rescue me.

I was in our kitchen. It was dinner time. Fran was so beautiful. She was gently stirring Papa Joe's homemade tomato sauce in a saucepan. I placed a baguette in the oven at three hundred degrees. I poured a glass of wine and took a sip as I set the table for two. Aabby, stretched out on the area rug like a sphinx, waited patiently near the dinner table. Fran sensed my eyes looking at her, turned, and smiled.

I suddenly cried out in pain. My reverie was broken. Gloria rushed to my side.

"What's wrong?"

I moaned. I gasped for air. I felt like I was going to heave. Another violent spasm. The Devil had entered my body. I needed an exorcist. I rolled over and grabbed hold of the steel bars on the side of my bed. Gloria rushed to get some help. Don't leave me alone. I think I might be dying. Gloria quickly returned with the night nurse, who urged me to take another pill for pain.

"No!" I shouted. "I don't want any more!"

I started writhing in bed like a wounded animal, unable to find any place of comfort.

"Please, Mr. Crystal. You must take something for your pain. It will help you sleep."

I gasped for air. A painful, relentless storm raged inside me. I was in the darkest depths of my own Katrina. My body convulsed wildly. Trying to hold on to something, anything – throw me a life raft! My levee suddenly broke and streams of salty tears washed my cheeks. I was going under, caught in a descending whirlpool. Sinking beneath the surface of my soul.

And then Julius, the male night nurse, entered the stormy night and stood beside me. He studied me briefly, then stroked my head with hands of calm assurance. He reached down and lifted me safely on my side. He steadied my ship with soft thick pillows. They were my sandbags. They anchored me. He talked to me, assuring me the storm would pass, and he would not leave my side until it did.

"Take the pill," he said calmly. "We only want to help you."

"Okay," I cried in surrender. "Give me the fuckin' pill."

The nurse handed me the pill in a small paper cup. Somehow, I managed to get it in my mouth. Gloria handed me a cup of ice water. I sucked on the straw and washed it down. I caught my breath. I tried to regain my focus. I looked at the concerned faces hovering around me. I had lashed out at the very people trying to help me. They didn't deserve to be treated that way.

"I'm sorry," was all I could say to them "for acting this way."

"Don't worry. It's alright. We understand."

And I knew they did. Julius had given me the courage to let go and come up for air. I stopped trembling. He was my bridge over troubled waters. A handsome, Filipino man, with the name of both my grandfathers, had come to rescue me. He asked for nothing. He expected nothing. His reward came from the smile that replaced the panic of pain I did not ask for nor deserve. He was my hero.

"You'll be okay," he said, touching me with his hand. He smiled and left quietly to rescue the next sinking stranger. I nodded off, my body exhausted from the violent interlude. I still couldn't sleep, even with the pill, but at least I could deal with it. It was suddenly two thirty in the morning. Gloria had been by my side every minute. She wiped my brow with a damp washcloth. That achy, feverish feeling was thankfully gone. The storm had passed.

"Wow," I told her. "I was in a very dark, scary place."

"You look better now. I think you should eat something."

"Really?"

"Yes. You need your strength."

"Okay. Fran left me some crackers. I just hope I don't throw up."

I cautiously started eating them. They tasted great. Gloria made me a cup of tea. Delicious. We talked between bites. I was having tea and crackers at three a.m. I began to grow sleepy. Gloria counseled me to fill my urine bottle before I nodded off. She propped up my pillow behind my head and made me feel comfortable. Before I knew it, I drifted off to sleep.

When I opened my eyes, it was a little after six a.m. Even though I had only slept three hours, I was full of energy, ready to start the day. I felt reborn. Gloria gave me a sponge bath and then said goodbye. She smiled when I thanked her for helping me through the terrible night.

"You're welcome," she said and left for home.

A member of Dr. Trento's staff came into my room to examine the drainage tube in my chest. The bleeding had stopped.

"Well, you won't be needing this anymore."

She removed it with a slight pull. No more drainage bag. No more anything. My body was completely intact.

"If all goes well, you could be going home tomorrow."

I was completely stunned. I reached for the phone. I knew it was early, but I had to tell Fran about this amazing turn of events. She's so relieved to hear me talking like myself again. She hadn't slept a wink. She's overjoyed that the drainage tube was now just a memory.

"Today's going to be a great day, Rip."

"Today is a great day," I replied with grateful energy.

"The kids are coming to visit later in the afternoon, and we're going to watch the Oscars." I couldn't wait.

I picked up the triflow and inhaled deeply. The first ball lifted up into the air like it had been shot out of a cannon. The second ball vibrated, like a strong breeze was passing by. Suddenly, miraculously, it leapt up into the air. I was filled with a sense of wonder and accomplishment. Nothing could stop me now. I was still holding my breath. I reached down for every bit of air in my body. The third ball quickly rose about half way up the chamber.

Oh, my God. I did it! I did it! I didn't know what to do next. Suddenly, I saw my iPod. I wanted to hear my music. I eagerly inserted my ear plugs and checked out my playlist. I yearned for Carmen MacRae. I stared out the window and gazed at the early morning sky. I was calm, serene. At peace with the world. And then, it began.

I can make out the muffled sounds of scattered jazz fans in some intimate late night bistro. Wine glasses tinkling occasionally. The deep warmth of a bass being plucked with a steady, calm pulse. A gentle brush kisses the circular canvas of a snare drum. Anxious anticipation fills the audience as they wait in hushed silence. She moves to the microphone with matronly grace. A quiet. And then, I hear her voice.

Carmen's rich caramel, coating my being with sweet elegance. Tickling my attentive ears. A breath. A pause. A graceful vocal dance on the melody ballroom floor. Mariah, Beyoncé, and Alicia sit at the foot of her throne. My eyes sparkle. My head nods knowingly in my hospital bed. Tears of appreciation flood my eyes. Although I had listened to Carmen's magical rendition of "My Foolish Heart" countless times, I had never really heard it until then. My body sways in time to the breeze of her voice. She invites me to join her. I can't resist. I open my throat. My soul sings.

"There's a line between love and fascination that's so hard to see on evening's such as this..." The moment transports me to pure joy.

***

Singing has always been my savior. My best friend. When I was lonely, it kept me company. When I was lost, it was my compass. It was my ticket to a summer in Banff, my passageway to the Kraft Music Hall, the vehicle that transported me to a career in the entertainment industry. It was the girlfriend that always loved me, no matter how many times I broke up with her.

After my brief success on the Kraft Music Hall, I continued to travel into New York and audition for jobs in the theatre. Time after time, I would be called back. But I never got the job. I grew tired of being rejected and didn't have the will to beat my head against the wall. And so I abandoned my singing career before it had a chance to get started. My Uncle Milt suggested working at a talent agency.

"I don't know if you'd be happy as an agent, Rip, but you'll see how it all works. It's a great way to earn a Master's Degree in show business."

It seemed like a good idea. Uncle Milt arranged an interview for me at the William Morris Agency on 55th Street and Sixth Avenue in Manhattan. At the time, William Morris was the most prestigious and powerful talent agency in the world. They were in a class by themselves.

A short time later, I was accepted into their agent trainee program at ninety dollars a week. At first, it was incredibly exciting. It was a whole new world. I met a lot of extraordinary people, many who became life-long friends. But, after my first year, the novelty of the job wore off, and I began to regret working there. I soon realized I had more talent than many of the people I was representing and felt I was living a lie. I missed singing so much that I taught myself how to play guitar just so I could accompany myself.

Another year went by. I grew more and more frustrated with the job, but I didn't know what else to do. One night, I was working for an attorney in the business affairs department and had to finish typing a lengthy contract. It was taking me forever. I was really pissed because I had to cancel a date with a girl I had just met.

I got up from my desk, walked down the long carpeted hallway, and disappeared into the men's room. I looked at myself in the mirror over the sink and suddenly began to sing. My big baritone voice bounced off the bathroom tile and surrounded me with sound. It was just the release I needed and put me back in touch with the inner me. As I made my way back down the hallway to return to my desk, a young woman assistant suddenly appeared from behind a partition. Her name was Vicki Vidal. Gore Vidal was a relative.

"Excuse me," Vicki asked politely. "Was that you singing?"

"Yeah, that was me," I admitted reluctantly.

"You have a beautiful voice," she said. "What are you doing here?"

I looked at her and simply replied, "I don't know."

"Listen, I've written a new musical and we're looking for a guy to join the cast and sing at a series of backer's auditions. Interested?"

That weekend I auditioned for Vicki and Sue Lawless, the show's director. I got the job. During the next six months, I sang in front of a live audience again and earned some extra money. Unfortunately, the show never found enough investors to get off the ground.

Another year passed. I was still stuck at William Morris, but my situation had greatly improved. I had been promoted to a junior agent and was making double my starting salary. I made deals for comedy duos Bob and Ray, and Jerry Stiller and Anne Meara. I sat in on pitch meetings, signed clients, and helped developed new projects. My future was bright.

And then, completely out of nowhere, I received an unexpected phone call. It was Sue Lawless, who directed me in the backer auditions. She asked if I had any interest in performing in a new musical revue she was traveling over the summer. It was an equity production and had a guaranteed run of six months.

I was moving up the ladder at William Morris but knew that, if I didn't seize the opportunity, I would regret it for the rest of my life. I was too young and too talented to give up on a singing career so soon. I raced over to her apartment during my lunch break and sang for the producers. They offered me the job on the spot. My voice had opened another door for me, and, with complete trust and faith in this fateful turn of events, I abandoned my promising career as an agent at William Morris.

I had a wonderful summer playing one of the leads in a musical revue called: "The Great American Fun Factory". It was a live musical variety show consisting of skits, blackouts, and song. Performing six nights a week gave me the opportunity to fine-tune my craft, find every little laugh, and connect with the audience more consistently. By the end of the run, I was on top of my game.

When I returned to New York, the reality of my new career hit me hard. I didn't have an office to go to, people to work with, and a paycheck at the end of the week. I was truly on my own, living on unemployment checks, searching the trades for my next job. I wasn't working nine to five anymore and had no idea what tomorrow would bring. But, I was confident that I had made the right decision and was fulfilling my destiny.

My new life style was invigorating. During the day, I would work on new songs, develop presentations for television shows, and ride the subway to my next audition. At night, I'd search local nightclubs and sing for free to showcase my talent and, hopefully, be discovered.

Months flew by. There were a lot of almosts, but nothing clicked. Unemployment was quickly running out, and I was going to have to do something to pay the rent. The fearful anxiety that led me to abandon my singing career some years before had returned again much sooner than I anticipated. I started doubting the wisdom of my decision to pursue my singing career but was determined to stick it out for as long as I could. I knew what I could do, and I wasn't going to quit.

A short time later, I received a call from Dulcy Eisen, a young woman I had met at William Morris who was now working at a small talent agency. A topical musical revue, which was having a successful run at Jimmy's, was looking for a versatile performer to replace one of the male leads. It was called: "What's a Nice Country like You Doing in a State like This?" I caught the show that night and knew instantly I was perfect for it. I absolutely nailed my audition and was hired to replace Gary Beach, a talented performer who would later win a Tony as the gay director in "The Producers".

I wasn't crazy after all. I was living the dream, making a living as an actor and a singer, appearing nightly in a hit show in New York. I stayed with the show for almost a year until it ended its run. People knew who I was now. I was hopeful that, before very long, I'd be singing on Broadway. But nothing came my way. I was back to square one, collecting unemployment, and looking for my next gig. It was tough to go through the insecurity and doubt again, but this was the life I chose, and I had nobody to blame but myself. But, again, just as my unemployment was running out, I auditioned to be the male understudy in the Broadway National Company of a musical revue called: "Nash at Nine" and was offered the job.

I didn't want to go on the road again, but I'd be working with director Martin Charnin, who wrote "Annie", and Milton Rosenstock, the musical director of "1776". It was the next step in my musical theatre career. I had toured in summer stock, appeared off-Broadway, and would now join the cast of a Broadway National Company. There was no way I could turn it down.

I only wish I had.

It was a complete and total disaster. Audiences didn't respond to the production at all. What made it even more humiliating was the fact that I never, ever got the opportunity to perform on the stage and work on my craft. It was the worst experience of my short career and left a bitter taste in my mouth. I returned to New York completely disillusioned, packed my bags, and flew to California with the dream of becoming the next Harvey

Korman on "The Carol Burnett Show." My timing couldn't have been worse. Television variety shows looking for singers like me were dead.

A few years later, after I began to make a living as a writer and producer, I abandoned my singing career again. I was now married to Fran, was a new dad, and owned a house. My priorities and circumstances had dramatically changed. But I never stopped singing. For friends and family, in the shower, in my car on the way to work. It was still my mistress, one of the great joys of my life.

After Mom passed away, I returned to Los Angeles and decided I wanted to record an album in her memory. She always wanted me to sing, and it was a way I could express my gratitude for her inspiration. I selected tunes that reflected the world I grew up in at the Commodore Music Shop and had meant so much to me.

I called the album "Nearer" in recognition of the Rodgers and Hart song I sang at her funeral. After I finished the album, I contacted Ahmet Ertegun in New York. Ahmet was a giant in the music industry and was very fond of my dad and Uncle Milt. I had met him some years earlier when I produced a documentary on the life of "Wild Bill" Davison, a Dixieland jazz cornetist that I knew from my childhood. I sent him the album and promptly received a note praising my selections and the beautiful way I interpreted them. I called him in New York and asked him if he knew of a record label that might be interested. He informed me that no one was going to sign an unknown, fifty-five year old singer who performed standards. The only way I could get my singing career off the ground was to perform again, build an audience, and create a buzz.

And so, after a twenty-five year hiatus, I decided to sing in public again. I made my debut at the Friar's Club in Los Angeles and really enjoyed it. A few months later, I sang at the Friar's in New York. People loved it. I was having a wonderful time. It was a great outlet for me. I was doing my thing. I didn't have to get notes from an arrogant young network executive or listen to my executive producer tell me that he didn't think my show was very funny. But, more importantly, it was a way for me to connect with my mom. Every time I sang, I felt she was listening and imagined her sitting in the back of the room with a big smile on her face.

Eventually, I developed a show called "When Jazz Was Pop". It featured songs of the 30's and 40's when jazz was America's popular music and gave me the opportunity to talk about the Commodore Music Shop and the musical legacy of my family. I was booked for two nights at Feinstein's at the Hollywood Roosevelt Hotel. The show was a wonderful success, and they invited me to perform it at their club in the Regency Hotel in New York.

The only night they had available was February 21st, 2004. I couldn't believe it. February 21st was the day of my Bar Mitzvah and coincidentally the day my parents got married. Word spread back East that I was going to be singing in New York, and the club was completely sold out. Many members of the audience were former classmates at Long Beach High. It was a great night.

Not long after that engagement, I received an email from Ellen Stauber, a former high school classmate. Ellen had heard about my performance in New York and was dying to hear me sing again. She was now living in Scottsdale, Arizona, happily married to Gene Schneller, a professor at Arizona State University. She asked me to put her on my email list and let her know when I'd be singing again in Los Angeles. It was a short flight from Scottsdale and her youngest son, Lee, had graduated from the University of Arizona and was now living in Westwood and working as a producer for the E cable network.

After some time, I developed a new show called "Soul to Soul". It featured the music of Harold Arlen and was scheduled to premiere at the Gardenia Supper Club in Hollywood on January 16th, 2006. Ellen called excitedly to tell me she was flying into town to hear me sing. She was hoping to bring her son and, because she didn't know anyone, asked if she could sit with Fran and Jackie. Fran was fine with the idea, but Jackie resented it. She thought it was a set up and didn't want to be manipulated. Lee didn't like the idea for two reasons. He was invited to attend the Golden Globes and didn't want to sit with the fat daughter of an old classmate of his mother's. But Ellen could be very persuasive and, somehow, managed to drag her resentful son to my show. Jackie didn't want to disappoint me and, reluctantly, agreed to sit at Fran's table.

Sparks were flying from the moment Jackie and Lee met. I don't think they heard one single note. This past September I sang at their wedding.

Many primitive cultures believe that the spirits of departed ancestors are always watching over us, protecting us, looking out for our best interests. I don't have any scientific data to support this conclusion, but I do know this. My mom adored Jackie. She was her youngest grandchild, an only child, and named for the love of her life. Mom was the reason I wanted to sing again, and, because I did, her granddaughter Jackie met the young man she would later marry.

I rest my case.

Chapter Fourteen
Oscar Night

Fran arrived early that morning and brought the Sunday paper. Needless to say, she was overjoyed to see me back among the living. We were equally excited that the kids were going to join us later to watch the Oscars. Fran had made four copies of the nominees that were listed in the calendar section of the L.A. Times so we could make our Oscar picks. It has been a ritual in our family for over twenty years.

My appetite was back in a big way. I made a point of drinking fluids as often as possible. I was about ready to take my morning stroll around the sixth floor when a nurse came into my room and informed me it was time to take an x-ray. A hospital attendant rolled in a wheelchair and helped me into it. When he ushered me outside, I saw Dr. Marty Gordon sitting at the nurse's station, accessing her computer. Marty happens to be my brother's doctor and we've been friends for years.

"So, how's it going?" he asked.

"It's a lot better now. Yesterday was intense."

"How many days after surgery?"

"Three days. The surgery was Wednesday."

"You hit the wall."

"What's that?"

"After the body is disrupted by a major surgery, it produces enormous amounts of adrenalin. It's a physical mechanism that helps you deal with the trauma. It usually takes a couple of days for the body to emerge from the shock. As it does, the adrenalin production returns to normal, and you crash from the loss of energy. We call it 'the wall'."

"Now you tell me."

Marty smiled. "You look great. You're going to be fine."

I smiled all the way to the elevator. As I sat with other patients in the holding area before being called to take my x-ray, I noticed an elderly man sitting in a wheelchair directly across from me. His shoulders were slumped dejectedly and his stubbled chin rested heavily against his chest. Upon hearing my arrival, he raised his head slowly. He was a pathetic figure, frail and sickly, with chalky white skin and a black patch over his left eye. His one eye looked out in my direction, helpless and disoriented.

**

I had seen that same look many years before on my father's face in Long Beach Memorial Hospital. He was sitting on a hospital bed wearing the very same black eye patch. He had been experiencing double vision and learned that he had arteriosclerosis, hardening of the arteries. Dad was frightened and didn't want me to see that he was. I remember hearing his bitterness when he angrily snapped at Mom, hurting her deeply.

Mom painfully replied, "I get the feeling you don't want me to be here."

Dad could only look away, realizing he had offended the woman that he absolutely adored.

When I think of my Dad, it is with remorse. I have always felt cheated that he didn't take care of himself and live a longer life. I know it isn't fair to blame him for his untimely death, but it left a huge black hole in my life that has never been filled.

Dad was a chain smoker, completely and totally addicted. He was part of the smoking generation, a generation that thought it was "cool" to smoke cigarettes. The fingers of his right hand were deeply discolored from the yellow stains of nicotine and tar – visible signs of the severity of his habit.

His brands of choice were Camels and Lucky Strikes. They were the real deal, sticks of dynamite without any filter. He would pound each new pack of cigarettes in his hand to compress the tobacco. But with each new smoke, no matter how hard he tried, he would still find himself removing small pieces of tobacco that would stick to the tip of his tongue. He was so hopelessly hooked that there were times when he would light a smoke, take a drag, and place it down in an ashtray. If he was distracted by a phone call or Mom asking for his help, he would forget that he had left a cigarette burning and light another one. It wasn't unusual to find ashtrays filled with the white flaky residue of cigarettes that had never been smoked.

When he'd step up to bat at a pickup softball game on a Sunday afternoon, he would need one of his boys to run to first base because he couldn't. It was always a struggle for Dad to climb the flight of stairs that led to the home of my Uncle Berns in Brooklyn. He frequently had to reach out for the banister and pause to catch his breath.

In January of 1964, three months after Dad's fatal heart attack, the Surgeon General publicly announced that smoking cigarettes was the main cause of the frightening rise of lung cancer and coronary disease. It infuriated me.

Jack Crystal was a bright man, extremely well educated. He was a graduate of St. John's Law School but never practiced. He earned his degree during the depression and firms weren't hiring. He ended up taking a retail sales job at Macy's in Manhattan. It was unfortunate he never fulfilled his potential, but he never regretted it. Because that's where he met my Mom.

He fell madly and desperately in love with her, but Mom wasn't sure if he was the one. Dad was from a poor working class family in Brooklyn. His mother, Sophie, was an uneducated seamstress and did the very best she could to provide for her family. Although a widow at a very young age, she never remarried. Dad was just sixteen when his father passed away. But, being the oldest child in the family, he quietly assumed the responsibility of helping his struggling mother and caring for his younger siblings, his brother, Berns, and sister, Marcia.

Mom was vivacious, talented, and beautiful. There never was a shortage of men at her doorstep, and she knew what she had to offer. She had dreams of her own and didn't know if Dad could make them come true. Dad was undeterred and pursued Mom relentlessly. He was extremely romantic and eventually convinced her that he could make her happy. They were married in 1939.

Unable to forge his own career, Dad went to work with his three brother-in-laws at my grandfather's music store in New York, The Commodore Music Shop. Originally a family hardware store, the music store was the visionary idea of my grandfather's first born, Mom's older brother, Milt Gabler. Dad was a proud man and was never one to take a handout. So he worked harder at the store than anyone else to prove to my Mom and her family that they were lucky to have him. And they were.

In the thirties and forties, The Commodore Music Shop was a New York institution. It was "the place" to buy records. There were feature magazine articles in Life, Cosmopolitan, and the New Yorker praising its remarkable success. In fact, it was so popular that Milt decided to produce his own records and created the Commodore Jazz Label. Eddie Condon, Jelly Roll Morton, Pee Wee Russell, George Brunis, "Wild" Bill Davison, and Willie "the Lion" Smith were just some of the giants of the jazz world who recorded for my Uncle Milt and Commodore. But his greatest triumph was undoubtedly the two albums he recorded with Billie Holiday. To this day, "Strange Fruit" is considered one of the most important recordings in the history of American popular music.

After the enormous success and notoriety of his recordings with Billie, Milt was recruited by Dave Kapp at Decca Records. He had no second thoughts about leaving the business he had created because he trusted and respected Dad so much. Milt became the Creative Vice President of Decca and remained there for thirty years. He recorded just about everyone, including Bing Crosby, Louis Armstrong, Ella Fitzgerald, Peggy Lee, Sammy Davis, Jr., The Andrew Sisters, Louis Jordan, Brenda Lee, The Mills Brothers, Burl Ives, and The Weavers. His recording of "Rock Around the Clock" with Bill Haley and the Comets changed the face of American popular music.

As Milt's career soared, Dad struggled to keep the Commodore Music Shop afloat. He poured his heart and soul into the business with the understanding that my grandfather would reward him with a stake in the company. But he never did. For all the years Dad worked at the Commodore Music Shop, he would never be more than a paid employee. It left him deeply resentful and bitter for the rest of his life.

His meager salary was barely enough to support his wife and three young sons. In order to make ends meet, he had to take on a second job. He began producing weekend jazz sessions at the Central Plaza, a catering hall on Second Avenue on the lower East Side, right next to Ratner's Restaurant and a neighborhood movie theatre, which later would become the legendary music hall, The Fillmore East. Every Friday and Saturday night, hundreds of college kids would pack the joint, listening to the hot music as they swallowed down pitchers of beer.

"Jazz at the Plaza" was Dad's thing. His love. His passion. But it was exhausting. No matter how late the sessions ran, Dad always made the hour drive home to Long Beach to sleep beside my Mom. I can never remember a night when he didn't.

Sadly, by the early fifties, people's tastes in music were quickly changing. Teenagers were listening to rock n' roll, dancing to Chuck Berry and Little Richard, and screaming at the revolutionary gyrations of Elvis Aaron Presley. Before long, Peter, Paul, and Mary, The Kingston Trio, and a nasally, wiry youth named Bob Dylan had begun to fill folk music clubs like "The Bitter End" in Greenwich Village.

And, if this wasn't enough pain for my father to endure, the record store was now losing money. The Commodore Music Shop was a boutique, a small family business that could no longer compete with the lower prices of Sam Goody's, a large retail record store that opened right around the corner. Against my father's wishes, my grandfather closed the shop in 1958. Dad was suddenly out of a job. When the decision was made to close the Commodore Music Shop, I was twelve years old. Dad drove us into the city to say goodbye. He told us to take some albums home as a memento.

The shelves were almost empty, but one striking album cover caught my attention. It was the photograph of a handsome, young black man holding his trumpet on his knee. For some reason, I was drawn to it. I briefly read the liner notes and scanned the titles of the tracks. They were all unfamiliar except for "Billy Boy". Grandma Susie loved to sing that song to my brother, so I decided to take it home.

The album was "Milestones". The trumpet player was Miles Davis. His incredible sextet featured two musicians I had never heard of - Cannonball Adderly and John Coltrane. When we returned home, I eagerly took out the LP and played it on the hi-fi in our living room. I was stunned. I had never heard anything like this before. It changed my life. I played the record constantly. When Dad witnessed my excitement as I listened to it, he became furious. I was forbidden to play the album when he was home. It served as a painful reminder that the traditional music that he loved was fading away, even in the world of jazz. Dixieland and swing were now considered old school. Screaming along with "The Saints Go Marchin' In" was not at all "hip" anymore. Dave Brubeck, Gerry Mulligan, Herbie

Mann, and Mongo Santamaria were what jazz fans were listening to now.

After the store shut down, things were really rough. Dad tried to find producing jobs, but they were hard to come by. I can only imagine the frightening thoughts that ran through his mind. How much longer can I do this? How can I afford to send three boys to college? How do I support my family when the industry I've made a living in is disappearing? The stress had to be overwhelming.

One night, two men came to the house who I had never seen before. My brothers and I wondered why Dad took them to the back bedroom. We soon found out. They were jazz collectors. Things had become so bleak that Dad was forced to sell his rare seventy-eight recordings to bring in some money. It was absolute agony to watch Dad show them to the door, their arms filled with his priceless records. He closed the front door behind them, paused quietly, then turned and walked back to his bedroom and shut the door. He never shared his pain – he was too proud for that. But he didn't have to. We could all feel it. A piece of Dad was gone with those rare records. He was never the same.

The last time I spoke with him was on a Tuesday evening. I was a freshman at the University of Bridgeport and usually called home on Sunday night when the rates were cheaper. But I couldn't wait for Sunday because I had great news. I had just landed a student aide position in the library. I'd be able to make some spending money and ease Mom and Dad's financial burden. Mom usually answered the phone, but, on this night, it was Dad. I shared my excitement about my new job.

"That's great, son," he simply said. I was proud of my accomplishment and to receive his praise.

"But if it takes away from your studies," he quickly added, "it isn't worth it. Don't worry about Mom and me. We'll figure it out."

I knew every dollar was a blessing, and it had to offer some relief. But Dad couldn't admit it. Three hours later, he died of a massive heart attack in the Long Beach Bowl.

For the first few years after his death, I resented him. He was the reason I had had to end my career at Bridgeport, live at home, and go to Brooklyn College at night. He was the man who couldn't provide for his family and deserted my Mom. It has now been over forty-five years since Dad passed away. Time has softened my anger, and I have sadly come to view him as a tragic figure. He never had the opportunity to enjoy his golden years with the woman he loved. He never saw his three sons marry girls from the neighborhood. Never felt the joy of bouncing one of his five grandchildren on his knee. He would have adored them.

I can't say I have totally forgiven him for his sudden exit. But, over the years, I've grown to appreciate the stress he was under, the desperate situation he found himself in, and the hollow feeling that gnaws at you when you live in the shadow of greatness and your accomplishments are overlooked.

***

A technician suddenly appeared in the holding area with a clipboard in his hand. He called my name, I raised my hand, and he wheeled me into x-ray. I struck two poses: front and side.

The young technician looked at the picture and exclaimed, "Man, you got long lungs."

"That's what years of playing woodwinds will do. Are they back to normal yet?"

"Just about. One lobe looks perfect. The other one isn't fully inflated. You should be good by tomorrow."

In a short while, I was back in my room and lunch was being served. The tall black attendant who was so gracious during my hellish Saturday, returned with Sunday's lunch tray. When he gently placed the tray down, I gave him a big smile.

"Don't I look a helluva lot better than yesterday?"

"I'm glad to see it," he said, shaking his head in joyful affirmation.

"Enjoy your meal."

"Thank you. I appreciate it."

He nodded politely and exited with a graceful bounce in his step. Billy stopped by to see how I was doing.

"I have something I want to show you," I said.

I took the triflow, inserted the plastic tube in my mouth, and sucked like a hoover vacuum. Almost instantly, the three balls exploded in the chamber. All he could say was, "Awesome." Fran was glowing. I smiled confidently with attitude and placed it down beside my bed.

We chatted briefly about the upcoming Oscar show. Billy was confident that Hugh Jackman would do a wonderful job as the host. As much as I enjoy Hugh and admire his talent, I still wanted to see Billy. Call me biased, but, in my estimation, there was never anyone better. Bob Hope and Johnny Carson were wonderful hosts, but limited to their charm and joke telling skills. Billy sang medleys, told jokes as well as anyone, and improvised brilliantly. And on top of all that, he would spend months in pre-production, putting together ingenious film pieces. They were remarkable and unforgettable. I wondered if he missed doing it again. Knowing my brother, I think he probably did.

Jackie and Lee stopped by soon after Billy said goodbye. Fran distributed the Oscar ballots, and we each picked our winners. I was totally into it. For the time being, I wasn't thinking about my health. What a pleasure.

As Billy predicted, Hugh did a wonderful job as the host, utilizing his musical talent and irresistible charm to maximum effect. Even though they tried to streamline the show, it was still too long. It would be the year that "Slum Dog Millionaire" came home with the golden statue time and time again. I loved the film, but felt the Oscar sweep was way overdone. More upsetting was the fact that the producers of the show failed to pay tribute to Paul Newman. No one deserved it more. Eventually the marathon show came to an exhausting conclusion. And guess what? Who do you think picked the most winners?

It was the perfect ending to a wonderful day. Soon, Fran and the kids said goodnight, and I was by myself. I took my meds and was hopeful the horror of the night before would only be a painful memory. I sat quietly in bed and rested peacefully. As I basked in the glow of my Oscar victory, I thought about my life-long love affair with the movies. I shook my head with a sense of wonder.

***

The city of Long Beach was blessed with a beautiful movie palace. It was a gold brick building on the southwest corner of West Park Avenue and Laurelton Boulevard. It was appropriately called the Laurel Theatre. It was a magnificent movie house, built in 1932. It had a seating capacity of two thousand with a balcony and a loge with comfortable seats.

When I was a kid, going to a movie was a major event. Like most families in Long Beach, we owned a small television and saw everything in black and white. So to be able to see a feature film on a huge screen in vibrant Technicolor was a thrill.

On Saturday mornings, the Laurel Theatre presented a children's matinee. Admission was twenty-five cents. There were cartoons, a Flash Gordon serial with Buster Crabbe, Three Stooges comedies, and a feature film. The theatre owners worked with the elementary schools in town and would distribute large cardboard tickets, about a foot long and two inches wide, for each Saturday matinee. They came in a variety of colors and were handed out randomly. When you arrived at the theatre early Saturday morning, a colored ticket would be taped to the glass paneled entry door. If the color of your ticket matched the color of the ticket that was posted, you gained free admission. We couldn't wait to get to the theatre and see if we had the winning color. It was always an exciting adventure.

The ticket booth was on the right hand side of the exterior lobby. The tiled floor was raked on an incline leading to a series of glass paneled doors. A matron, dressed appropriately in costume, would take your ticket, tear it in half, and hand you the stub. Once inside, there was a softly lit, plush carpeted lobby with upholstered arm chairs. Without much difficulty, you could hear the soundtrack of the film playing inside the theatre as you stood before a large, lengthy concession stand that sold soda, candy, and popcorn. At either end of the concession stand were two aisleways that led uphill into the theatre. When you stepped inside, you stood on a carpeted floor at the back of the raked orchestra section. A low metal railing acted as a border behind the very last row. If you turned around with your back to the screen, you would face a plush loge section and, beyond that, a huge balcony.

The Laurel Theatre had continuous screenings. Oftentimes, you could see double features. I never worried about what time a movie began. I loved to sit down to watch a movie from the middle. I'd see it through to the ending then sit through previews, newsreels, and anything else that was being screened. I'd then watch the movie again - from beginning to end.

My first movie memory was a scary one. I was six years old, an impressionable first grader, seeing "The Wizard of Oz" for the very first time. I was on the edge of my seat as the menacing Kansas wind kicked up and howled forcefully. Dorothy was rushing home to seek shelter from the storm, but the wooden doors that lead to the basement had been locked. For protection, she raced into her home with her little dog, Toto, cradled in her arms. The tornado struck with full force, and the house was lifted into the sky. Cows and chickens flew past Dorothy's bedroom window. It all seemed harmless enough. Then, the evil Mrs. Gulch appeared, peddling her bicycle in mid-air.

Suddenly, completely by surprise, Mrs. Gulch, accompanied by a harrowing melody, morphed into a wicked witch riding on her broomstick. Her maniacal laugh scared the hell out of me. I was so frightened that I literally jumped out of my seat. In a complete panic, I crouched down behind the seat in front of me, praying the wicked witch wouldn't see me. Years later, in the very same theatre, I'd have another harrowing experience watching the horrific finale of Alfred Hitchcock's "Psycho". I didn't hide behind the seat in front of me, but I was completely freaked out. Never in a million years did I think Tony Perkins and his mother were the same person. Genius.

I saw Danny Thomas in "The Jazz Singer", Doris Day and Rock Hudson in "Pillow Talk", Burt Lancaster and Jean Peters in "Apache". Marlon Brando telling his brother Charlie 'he coulda been a contenda' in "On the Waterfront". A teary Montgomery Clift playing taps for Frank Sinatra in "From Here to Eternity". A tormented Warren Beatty leaving broken-hearted Natalie Wood behind in "Splendor in the Grass". The brilliant James Dean desperate for his father's love in "East of Eden". A young Paul Newman sitting on the hood of an open convertible, waving to cheering fans after winning the championship as boxer Rocky Graziano in "Somebody Up There Likes Me". That film had special meaning to people in Long Beach because Rocky lived in town, and you could see him every Sunday morning buying the paper at the Cozy Nook luncheonette. I experienced the epic spectacles of "The Robe", "Demetrius and the Gladiators", "The Ten Commandments", and the amazing chariot race in "Ben Hur".

Musical movies were a special treat for me. Fred Astaire adoring Audrey Hepburn in "Funny Face", Gene Kelly in his baseball cap, white socks, and penny loafers dancing for giggling kids in Paris to "I Got Rhythm", Susan Hayward as legendary singer Jane Froman courageously entertaining the troops after a crippling plane crash in "With a Song In My Heart", Yul Brynner as the proud King of Siam uttering 'et cetera, et cetera, et cetera' in "The King and I", Jimmy Stewart blowing into a trombone as Glen Miller, Danny Kaye as Red Nichols making his comeback at the end of "The Five Pennies", Bing Crosby and Satchmo singing "Now You Has Jazz" in "High Society", Russ Tamblyn doing back flips in "Seven Brides for Seven Brothers". Oh God, I could go on and on.

To think that this impressionable kid from the small town of Long Beach on the south shore of Long Island would somehow end up in Hollywood decades later and produce a major motion picture starring Sandra Bullock completely blows my mind. But the most meaningful memory I have in the Laurel Theatre had nothing to do with movies.

On the 23rd of June in 1963, the Laurel Theatre was the site of my high school graduation. I was asked to sing a stirring art song called "The Trumpeter", by J. Airlie Dix. I was accompanied on an acoustic piano by a young woman I had known since elementary school, Gari Zerfuss. Without a microphone, my baritone voice filled the enormous hall. As I looked out at the sea of loving friends, family, teachers, and leaders of the community, I realized that my voice had been chosen to express the soul and spirit of my classmates. It was thrilling and, indeed, humbling.

This was a special moment. It was more than just a song. It was a thank you from a grateful young man to a community that had watched him grow, supported, and nurtured him. That cheered him at basketball games, had him over for dinners at their houses, and made him feel part of an extended family. After I held the final note and Gari struck the last chord on the piano, I stood in a moment of silence. Momentarily, a wave of applause engulfed me and swept me off the stage to rejoin my classmates.

It was a beautiful farewell.

***

I looked down remorsefully at the hospital floor. Regretfully, the magical, magnificent Laurel Theatre was closed in the early seventies, not even ten years later. It was a terrible loss. It should have been preserved as a historical landmark. Now, it only remains as a priceless memory to those who experienced it and a sad reminder of a community that lacked vision.

Suddenly, my head snapped up with a burst of hopeful energy. My bitterness and regret was quickly replaced by an incredible realization. "Holy shit," I thought to myself. "This could be my last night in the hospital. I might be going home tomorrow."

Chapter Fifteen
Then Came You

I was awakened from a restful sleep just minutes after four a.m. It began with a mild rumbling below my belly button. My body was sending me an alert. After five long days, the time had come. Somewhat groggy from a sleeping pill, I cautiously sat up and dangled my feet over the side of the bed. I looked down. After a short moment of visual scanning, I located my slippers. I slid down off the bed and placed my feet inside them. I used my arms to gently but firmly push my body upward until I was standing on my feet. I could see the light filtering onto the floor from inside the bathroom door. I moved towards it – one small step at a time.

I reached the door and slowly opened it. I stepped inside the bathroom and closed the door behind me. I looked down and studied my porcelain target. Hovering above it, I turned slowly, took a breath, and bent my knees. As I lowered my body, I focused my weight on the large quadricep muscles in my thighs. I extended my long arms towards the floor and placed my hands on the sides of the drop zone for support. I cautiously eased my body down, paused anxiously for a brief moment, and then made my final descent.

I smiled with a sense of accomplishment. I had made a perfect landing. I closed my eyes and tried to relax. There was another brief rumble emanating from my lower intestine. I was advised not to force the issue and just let nature do what it's supposed to. Nature didn't let me down. It was perfection. All systems were go. I sighed with relief as my body cleansed itself. It was absolutely fantastic.

There was no way I could sleep. I picked up one of Jackie's crossword books, put on my reading glasses, armed myself with a ballpoint pen, and started with one across. I love crossword puzzles and the challenge they present to my intellect. I can't start the morning without opening the paper and taking one on. To me, it's mental gymnastics. Aerobics for the mind. Besides expanding my vocabulary and teaching me about people, places, and things, it has taught me the value of persistence, patience, and trust.

This has happened to me time and time again. I have most of the puzzle solved except for one small section. If I can find the answer to a key question that connects all the other words, everything else will fall into place, and I'll have another win on my crossword scorecard. I look at the remaining blank spaces from every angle I can think of. I focus all my energy on trying to solve it. But, try as I may, I just can't figure it out.

I'm getting tense. My mind is freezing up. In the past, I'd throw in the towel and admit defeat. But that is no longer the case. I have learned that, if I trust my intellect, stick with it, and remain confident, the answer will eventually come. So, I would leave the puzzle alone, finish my breakfast, wash the morning dishes, and start my day. Sometime later, it could be lunchtime, dinnertime, or before going to bed, I return to the puzzle and try again. And, voila, just like that, I see the question from a different perspective and, inevitably, come up with the correct answer. It never ceases to amaze me.

So now, as I probed my mind and filled in the blanks, I began to grow tired. My eyes felt heavy, and I dozed off to sleep. I awoke sometime after six and proudly told the morning nurse that I had finally gone to the bathroom. She congratulated me. I was anxiously awaiting the arrival of a member of Dr. Trento's team. She came sometime after eight. She looked at the incision and the site where she removed my drainage tube.

"So, what's the verdict?" I asked anxiously.

"I spoke with Dr. Trento this morning and went over your numbers. Everything looks very good. You'll be going home today."

"That's so fantastic."

"Someone from the office will go over everything before you leave. We'll see you in about ten days to remove the stitches. Okay?"

"Absolutely."

She smiled routinely, turned, and simply walked away. Like Dr. Trento had said when I first met him, "I know it's a big deal for you, but we do this all the time." And then I remembered the words of Dr. Kedan after I listened to my new heart in critical care.

"I won't be back until Tuesday. You'll probably be home by then." Right again.

I was so excited. I had no second thoughts about the decision. I was ready to go home. I reached for the phone and called Fran. She was in the supermarket, doing a big shop, preparing for my return.

"Have you heard anything?"

"Great news," I said excitedly. "Frannie... I'm coming home today."

Fran screamed with joy. And then, I started to choke up.

"I'm sorry, honey. It's just such a relief."

Fran started to cry. "I need you to be strong for me," she said. For the first time since this ordeal began, Fran let her guard down, revealing the tension she didn't want me to see. She had been so supportive from the very beginning, always positive, always reassuring me whenever I expressed my fears and anxiety.

"I love you, Fran."

"And I love you."

When I hung up the phone, I thanked my lucky stars for this beautiful soul, this dear, dear woman who, on one fateful Saturday morning in 1975, walked off a plane in the Los Angeles airport and changed my life forever.

***

It was July. I was lying on a two-inch piece of foam covered in a black sheet that served as my bed in the living room of the one-bedroom apartment I shared with Joel Gotler. Joel and I met when we worked together at the William Morris Agency in New York in the early seventies. He was a soulful, brilliant guy who loved books and played a great blues harmonica. I was a frustrated performer who loved to strum my guitar and sing. We totally connected. In April, I had returned to New York City after traveling on the road with the National Company of "Nash at Nine". The girl I was living with had met someone else.

I called Joel, who had moved to L.A. He was working at Universal Studios as the assistant to legendary producer, Jennings Lang. After filling him in on my misery, Joel insisted I come out west and live with him. He had this cool little house he was renting in Beverly Glen and there was plenty of room. In less than one week, I was on a plane to the coast. I would never look back.

Joel met me at the airport in Los Angeles with another transplanted William Morris colleague, Elliot Webb, who was working as a young television agent at ICM. And, just like that, I was in L.A., ready to roll the dice on a career in show business. It was a huge rush. Anything was possible. After a couple of months, the lease on the house in Beverly Glen expired. Elliot helped Joel and I find a one bedroom apartment in his building in Beverly Hills.

So, early on a particular Saturday morning in July of 1975, the doorbell rang. It was Elliot. He was emotionally distraught. A girl he met while attending an intensive training weekend called EST, created by Werner Erhard, had completely rejected him. He was in a lot of pain. He asked if I could keep him company as he drove to the airport to pick up his sister, Carol, who was flying in from New York. I hemmed and hawed but felt for the guy. The pain of being rejected by a woman was a feeling I knew only too well and decided to take the ride. It was the best decision I ever made.

Elliot and I approached the gate to wait for his sister, Carol. It was before 9/11 and security wasn't an issue. As he went on about his emotional pain and the woman who broke his heart, I recognized Kate Remo and Alice Flax, two young women from my hometown of Long Beach, standing nearby. We had a brief conversation to catch up on our lives. I soon learned that Kate and Alice were both living in Los Angeles and were waiting for their childhood friend, Frannie Agovino. Fran would be spending three weeks vacationing in California before returning to her apartment in Queens and her teaching job that would start up again in September.

"Do you remember, Frannie?"

I vaguely did. All I knew about their friend was that she was in my brother's class and she was the girlfriend of John Candeleria, a good-looking, talented basketball player.

The plane arrived. Passengers began to filter into the terminal.

And then I saw her.

She was dressed smartly in a black top and white slacks. She was the epitome of a classy, young, New York woman, an absolute knockout. Her hair was thick, black, and was neatly styled to the nape of her tapered neck. She had a beautiful figure, graceful and firm, and walked with an air of calm assurance. When her face lit up and her eyes sparkled at seeing her childhood girlfriends, she reminded me of a young Natalie Wood.

We shared a brief hello. Fran was somewhat stunned to see me. As it turned out, she had been walking on the sands of Long Beach the day before and ran into my brother, Billy, his wife, Janice, and their little baby, Jenny. When Billy learned Fran was traveling to Los Angeles to visit Kate and Alice, he told her I had just moved out there. After Fran said goodbye, Billy turned to Janice. "We should have given Fran Rip's number. They'd make a great couple."

But he never did. It was an amazing coincidence. I looked deeply into Fran's sparkling brown eyes and felt like I was home. I had never felt anything like that before. Alice and Kate invited me to join them for dinner in the valley the following night. I said I'd love to.

As Elliot and I drove Carol back to his apartment, she informed us she was lucky to get a seat on the plane. Someone had cancelled their reservation at the last minute. That Sunday night, we ate outdoors in Alice's backyard, shared a glass of wine, and reminisced about growing up in Long Beach. And then I learned that Fran almost cancelled her trip. Her friend from New York, Julie, was scheduled to travel with her. She had met a guy in the city, fallen in love, and decided not to come at the last minute.

"Oh, my God," I said. "You won't believe this." Everyone turned to look at me in anticipation. "Elliot's sister may have gotten Julie's seat."

Very powerful forces in the universe were at work here. How else could you explain this mystical connection? Something magical was happening. I couldn't take my eyes off her. I smiled. She tilted her head and smiled back. That was all the encouragement I needed. I got up from my seat, walked to her side, and whispered, "Let's get out of here. I want to be alone with you." She looked up at me warmly and simply said, "Okay."

Fran slid into the passenger seat of my 1967 black mustang convertible. I put the top down, turned on the radio, and headed off for scenic Coldwater Canyon. The southern California breeze was invigorating. We didn't have to say very much. I was pretty sure we were feeling the same thing. We drove down Sunset Boulevard to take in the striking billboards on the strip. Everything was aglow. It was a beautiful night. We ended up in Hollywood and walked the boulevard together. Like most tourists, we pointed out the Hollywood stars embedded in the pavement and shared stories about our past.

It was at the corner of Hollywood and Vine. The light turned red and we paused. It was my cue. I reached over and gently took her hand. She looked up at me with sparkling eyes. I slowly leaned down and kissed her.

We spent that first sleepless night together in Kate's apartment, locked in each other's arms. Fran and I had found what we'd been looking for and were making sure it wouldn't get away. For the next three weeks, we were inseparable. Within forty-eight hours, we were driving up the coast on our way to San Francisco. Dionne Warwick and the Spinners sang, "*I never knew love before, then came you, then came you.*" We stopped for a hamburger in Big Sur, walked the pier in Monterrey, and hung out in Golden Gate Park.

It was so incredibly joyous, so magical, so romantic. Although we had both been hurt in the past and were tentative to expose our feelings once again, we trusted our instincts and surrendered to each other completely. Before we knew it, our unforgettable three weeks together came to a close. We were back in the airport terminal where we had first met. Only now, we were saying goodbye.

Fran looked up at me with a tear in her eye and said, "It was great, Rip."

That's all. I looked down at her and told her this was not the end to our relationship but the beginning. Only time would tell. We wrote letters, spoke on the phone at least once a week, and grew to trust each other even more. This was special. We began to make plans. Fran had her degree in special education, taught Braille, and worked with the visually impaired in New York. She contacted the Los Angeles School District and set up an interview with the administrator of her specialty. Without much difficulty, she was offered a teaching position in Los Angeles. We were right on schedule. I made plans to fly to New York for Christmas and New Year's. We couldn't wait to be together again. The morning I was scheduled to leave, I received a phone call from Elliot Webb, who was now working with me and representing some of my projects.

"Great news, Rip," he said excitedly. "Ted Kotcheff thinks you might be right for a scene in a new comedy feature: "Fun with Dick & Jane". They want to see you today."

I didn't want to be bothered with another painful audition. All I wanted to do was get to New York and be with Fran.

"Elliot," I said. "I'm leaving for New York at three o'clock. Is there any chance we can do it when I come back?"

"Ripper, listen to me. Don't be a schmuck. It's with George Segal and Jane Fonda. There'll be another flight."

I reluctantly took his advice and made the audition. As I waited in the casting office, I was a bundle of nervous energy. I kept looking at the clock on the wall and wondered if I could still make my flight. After an interminable wait, my name was finally called. Ted asked me to read the scene a couple of different ways, smiled, and thanked me for the audition. It was over in a matter of minutes.

I sped to the airport in the hope I could still make my flight, but there was no way. Traffic was completely backed up. It was a Christmas vacation nightmare. I desperately tried to get on another plane, but all the direct flights to New York were booked. Not one freakin' seat. I was so pissed. The audition was a waste of fucking time. I knew I shouldn't have listened to Elliot. There was nothing I could do about it now except figure out some way to get to New York. I pleaded my case to a friendly airline employee. She miraculously managed to get me on a late afternoon plane to Las Vegas. I eventually connected to a plane that got me to New York and reunited me with my soul mate.

I stayed with Fran in her apartment in Queens. It was a small one-bedroom and was tastefully decorated. She was neat and organized, like I was. I was comfortable. I belonged there. She cooked for me, she laughed with me, she loved me. She introduced me to her parents Joe and Belle and how an Italian family celebrates Christmas. It was wonderful. There was Joe's sister, Anna, Aunt Clara, and cousin Babe. I talked sports with cousins Sal and Vinnie, while Fran shared childhood memories with their wives. I met Lucretia and Mark and Minnie Romeo, from Metuchen, New Jersey, who had shining eyes and more energy than a woman half her age. It was a loving family that absolutely adored Fran. They were so happy for us both.

And the food. My God. I thought Grandma Susie was a great cook. I savored homemade tomato sauce, baked ziti with ricotta, eggplant parmigiana, mouth-watering braciola, and tasted Joe's amazing lobster fra diavolo for the very first time. There were cannolis, biscotti, and holiday pudding. All I kept hearing the entire vacation was, "You want another glass of wine? Eat, Rip, eat. Mangia." I felt right at home.

Fran got to meet Joel and Barbara and their young children, Jonathan and Faithe. We all went to Carnegie Hall and joined Janice to cheer for Billy when he opened for Melissa Manchester. I was still a bachelor. Living on my own. My brothers were both married to great, hometown girls. They were having so much fun raising their families. I envied their good fortune. Fran changed all that.

California was the furthest thing from my mind when I suddenly received a phone call one December night in Fran's apartment. It was Elliot Webb to tell me congratulations. Ted Kotcheff wanted me for his movie. Shortly after I returned to L.A., on one unforgettable winter night, I shot the scene with George Segal and Jane Fonda in a motel on Sunset Boulevard. It was absolutely amazing. Everything was coming together.

And then I got a call from my brother Joel in Long Beach. He had just gotten off the phone with my first love, Cheryl. She saw Billy on "The Tonight Show" and wanted to get in touch with me. She was happily married and had moved to Fresno, California. When she learned I was living in Los Angeles, she couldn't believe it. She would definitely be giving me a call. My heart started beating faster. She was still thinking about me...

I first saw Cheryl on a Saturday afternoon at the Recreation Center near Reynolds Channel in Long Beach. Besides the beach, the boardwalk, and the outdoor basketball court at Central School, the "Rec" was one of the major hangouts for teens in town. There were bumper pool tables, ping pong, and music playing the latest songs we heard on "American Bandstand". The girls and the guys did their own thing and sort of checked each other out.

It was the spring of my junior year in high school. This particular afternoon, there were a group of young girls from the freshman class, my brother's class, eyeing some of the older boys. She was wearing black slacks with a short red jacket that hung just above her waist. It reminded me of the jacket that matador's wear in the bullring. She had olive skin and long blonde hair that cascaded down her back, like strands of gold. She moved with an effortless grace and sensual elegance that took my breath away. Quite simply, she was absolutely stunning. The most beautiful young woman I had ever seen.

I remember coming home that afternoon and asking Billy if he could give me any info. Her name was Cheryl Straus. She was dating a guy that was actually a year older than me, so timing might be a problem. I left it alone. And then, one day at school, as I was just about to open a door and enter the music room to make a jazz band rehearsal, Cheryl appeared right before me. She was leaving a choir rehearsal. Our eyes met. She smiled.

"Hi," I said.

"Hi," she replied.

I turned and watched her walk down the corridor to make her next class. I couldn't get her out of my mind. I was hooked. I finally got up the nerve to ask her out for a date, and, to my surprise, she said yes. We caught a movie at the Laurel Theatre with Bobby Wellen and his girlfriend, Roni. When I sensed the time was right, I reached over and took her hand. She didn't pull away. She caressed mine. And that's how it began. I was head over heels in love. Everything I did took second place to being with her. I had to be with her. She was all I ever thought about. We couldn't keep our hands off each other. The sexual chemistry between us was combustible. Sparks were everywhere.

She lived just a few short blocks away. On Sundays, her parents would drive to Queens to visit her grandparents. She would tell them that she couldn't make the trip, that she had to study for a test. The moment they drove away, she'd call me. I'd race over to be with her, and we'd spend the rest of the afternoon in bed.

Cheryl and I lost our virginity in my senior year. It was New Year's Eve. Her parents were out for the evening to celebrate the arrival of 1963, and her kid brother was finally asleep. My heart was beating like a hummingbird. I didn't know what I was doing. There was no sex education, no parent talk about the birds and the bees, no advice from a friend. But the time had come, and, somehow, we figured it out. She now had me completely.

I gave her my varsity jacket and bought her an ankle bracelet with our names on it. Her parents let us borrow their silver Buick Riviera so that we could go to the Prom in style. I was consumed by her. We agreed to see other people while I was away at school. With me out of the picture, I knew that guys would be lining up to ask her out. And, sooner or later, she would say yes. So I chose the University of Bridgeport. Cheryl was only a two hour drive away.

My mom's cousin, Al Shedler, was a successful CPA in Manhattan. He represented stage actors Jason Robards, Jr., Gloria Foster, Diana Sands, and the Circle in the Square. He was a great guy and wanted to bring me into his business. So I decided to major in accounting. I'd make a good living, and Cheryl's parents would approve. I had it all figured out. My future was guaranteed. And then, just two short months after I started school in Connecticut, my father died of a heart attack.

Cheryl's parents were sympathetic to my situation, but insisted she continue to see other people while I finished my freshman year at Bridgeport. Cheryl rebelled against their wishes and refused to date anyone else. I was the guy she wanted to spend the rest of her life with. Or so I thought.

The first time Cheryl broke my heart was during my recovery from kidney surgery in June of 1964. I was in the hospital for most of the month. The aura of being one of the most popular kids in high school had quickly vanished. Cheryl would spend the summer at the Malibu Beach Club in Lido Beach. She had the figure of Donna Michelle, the Playmate of the year, and wore beautiful bikinis her mother had bought her in Paris. Towards the end of the month, her visits to the hospital became less frequent. She seemed quiet. Unresponsive. I knew something wasn't right. I called her and asked her what was going on.

She simply said, "I met someone at the beach club."

I was utterly devastated. I was emotionally and physically defenseless. But my family and friends rallied around me, and, somehow, I managed to survive. I got healthy very soon. And, by a strange coincidence, one of my friends got me a job as a Cabana Boy at the Malibu, Cheryl's beach club. I didn't know if I could handle seeing Cheryl and her new boyfriend on a daily basis, but I sucked it up and took the job. I really didn't have a choice. It was a great opportunity to make some serious money. I played it cool.

Didn't push anything. Didn't act like an asshole. I'd say hello. Nothing more. After a while, Cheryl and I began to spend more time together. Nothing serious. Just brief conversations. She seemed interested.

And then Bobby Wellen called to let me know he had two tickets to see Johnny Mathis in concert at the stadium in Forest Hills. We could double. It sounded great, but I didn't know who to ask.

"Why don't you ask Cheryl?" he said.

"What? Are you out of your fucking mind?"

"What do you have to lose? She can only say no."

I was scared shitless but summoned up the courage to ask Cheryl to be my date. To my surprise, she said she'd love to. As we listened to Johnny sing "Chances Are", Cheryl reached over and grabbed my hand. I breathed a sigh of relief. I turned and looked into her eyes. Under the summer starlit night, listening to Johnny Mathis, we kissed once again. I felt her warmth on my lips. It melted me. I knew I had won her back. That night, I asked her to end the relationship that had come between us. She said she would break it off the next time she saw him.

That night came. I was so anxious I couldn't stand it. Compelled by my insecurity, I borrowed my Mom's white Dodge Lancer and drove by her house. My timing couldn't have been more perfect. The porch light was on and I could see him make his way out the door. His head was down, and I knew she had ended it. I was so relieved. And then, suddenly, Cheryl appeared in the doorway behind him. She reached up and lovingly wrapped her arms around his chest in a tender embrace. Adrenaline raced through my body. I swallowed hard and continued past her house. I drove for a couple of blocks then had to park the car. I was stunned and had to get my head straight. True, Cheryl broke it off and chose me. But now I had to live with this image in my head and the knowledge that she clearly had deep feelings for someone else.

Cheryl was now a senior at Long Beach High School. I was living at home, attending Brooklyn College at night. Within a few months, she began sending out college applications. She briefly considered living at home and attending Hofstra or Adelphi. Her parents insisted she should have the experience of going away to school and meeting new people. I hated to admit it, but I knew they were right. She would go to Boston University.

Every day I would greet the mailman hoping to hear from her. The letters came almost daily. As the days crept by, the letters came less frequently. The occasional phone calls much, much briefer. She was drifting away, but I was hopeful we'd get things back on track when I saw her in Boston for Homecoming Weekend. She never gave me the chance.

The night before I was to leave for Boston, my bags already packed, Cheryl called to tearfully tell me she had met an older guy who simply swept her off her feet. She struggled to get the words out. She didn't want to hurt me. I had meant the world to her. I then asked her if she was going to marry the guy, hoping this new relationship was only a brief affair, an impressionable, vulnerable young girl's momentary lack of judgment.

She simply said, "We've talked about it."

Those words hit me right in the gut with the power of a Marciano body shot. I crumbled.

"I'll always love you," she cried tenderly.

All I could say was, "I hope you're happy."

I hung up the phone as tears filled my eyes. I ran the water in the kitchen sink and washed the streams of salt that had reddened my cheeks. Billy was away at Marshall University, and it was just Mom and me. I staggered into her bedroom and told her what had happened. Mom knew my pain. She tried to console me, but only time would heal my wound.

"You're young. You have your whole life ahead of you. When you least expect it, the right girl will come along."

In some ways, I was relieved. After seeing Cheryl's embrace on her front porch, I knew it was just a matter of time. It was done. I didn't live in a state of lover's limbo anymore. I tried to get on with my life. I did the best I could. When the kitchen phone would ring, shattering the nighttime stillness, I secretly hoped it might be her. I'd rush to the mailbox with the youthful expectation she'd write of her confusion, her vulnerability, her regret. The letter never came. Life went on. It had been two years since the break-up. I felt no passion, just going through the motions. And then I took Dr. White's speech class and everything changed.

I literally found my voice and life was filled with hope and infinite possibilities. I was now a theatre major, singing my heart out. I made it home late one night after a rehearsal and turned the light on in the kitchen. I looked up at the blackboard on the wall and caught my breath. All it took was two little words scribbled in white chalk to get my heart racing.

"Cheryl called."

I knew it was late, but I couldn't wait. I reached for the phone and dialed her number. I had never forgotten. She answered the phone. She knew it was me. She sounded so happy. We made small talk and caught up on the events of our lives. That older guy who swept her off her feet was now a thing of the past. It felt great to talk to her again, to hear her voice. Right before we said goodnight, to my utter and complete surprise, Cheryl asked me a simple question that only I could answer.

"Would you like to go the movies, Rip? There's a picture I want you to see."

It was early winter. A light snowstorm hit New York as we waited on line outside the movie theatre on the upper east side of Manhattan. The picture was "The Graduate". I was sitting in the theatre with the girl of my dreams, watching a movie about a young guy who, at all costs, fights to be with the girl of his dreams. This was either a cruel, sadistic trick or a tender, loving message of reconciliation. Knowing Cheryl as well as I did, it had to be the latter. After the film, we took the Long Island Railroad from Penn Station back to Long Beach. The snow continued to fall. The train was practically empty. Cheryl took off her shoes, grabbed hold of my arm, and snuggled up beside me.

That beautiful white winter night, Cheryl and I made love again in the den of our house on East Park Avenue. She returned to school in Boston. We spoke on the phone more frequently now. I made sure to keep my emotional distance as a means of self-protection. The scars ran much too deep. She was home for Spring Break, and we spent the day in Central Park. We were sitting on the grass, sharing a picnic lunch. There was a tense pause in our conversation. She looked up at me and simply said, "Rip, I love you. I've always loved you. I can't stop thinking that we should get married."

"Seriously?" I said.

"I think about it all the time."

I was in shock. I didn't know what to say or how to react. Wasn't this what I wanted? Weren't these the words that I dreamed of hearing? But damn it, I couldn't commit. How could I trust her? She had broken my heart twice, and who was to say she wouldn't do it again. Sure enough, the summer after her college graduation, she was working on Wall Street, met a young man from France, and ran away with him. Her love affair quickly ended. She returned to New York and enrolled as a psychology major at the New School for Social Research. The last time I had spoken with her, she was involved in a serious relationship, and I was living with someone in New York. As time passed, I had rarely thought about her since I had moved to L.A. and fallen in love with Fran.

The moment of truth came that spring. Fran was on her Easter Break. She flew to Los Angeles to be with me and sign her contract for her special education teaching position that would begin in September. We had excitedly unpacked her furniture she had shipped from New York and were getting our apartment ready. We spent the day at Venice Beach with Roger Rexer, a friend of mine from San Francisco who happened to be visiting L.A. When we returned to my apartment, there was a familiar voice on my answering machine. It was Cheryl. She was coming to L.A. for a business conference and wanted to see me.

Fran turned white. This was not the faceless voice of some old girlfriend innocently calling to say hello. She knew Cheryl. They were in the same class in Long Beach High. She had pictures in her head of the two of us together. This was more than just a friendship. Something had to be going on if we were still in touch after all these years.

Fran made her stand. There couldn't be any if's. She was uprooting her life, moving across the country to be with a struggling actor. She had too much self-respect to make that kind of commitment to someone who might be having second thoughts. She angrily gave me an ultimatum.

"I don't want you to speak to her again. If you do, I'm leaving."

Fran turned abruptly and walked out of the apartment. I was speechless. Roger knew what was at stake and didn't want me to fuck up my life.

"Rip, Fran is the best thing that ever happened to you. You guys are meant to be together. She's you're future. Cheryl's your past."

"I know that."

"Do you love Fran? Really love her."

"Of course I do."

"Then call Cheryl and end it."

I knew he was right. I picked up the phone and returned Cheryl's call. I told her that I was in love with Fran and that our staying in contact made her extremely uncomfortable. Cheryl was disappointed but understood. I found Fran outside on the verge of tears. I told her I had called Cheryl and told her it was over. We embraced. My love for Fran was real. She was the woman I had been waiting almost ten years for. The right woman my mother told me would come along that painful night in her bedroom.

In the early part of July, Fran packed up her blue Chevy Nova in New York and drove cross country with Lenny Remo, Kate's younger brother. That summer, a year after we met, we were sitting with Billy and Janice on the beach in Santa Monica.

Billy simply said, "Why don't the two of you get married?"

Billy could sense my anxiety. He knew I was struggling to get my career off the ground.

"It doesn't have to be a big deal. You could tie the knot in our apartment."

Now I was really on the spot.

"I guess we could do it over the Christmas vacation. I'm sure Mom will make it, and Joel and Barbara would be on a break from teaching... Does that sound good to you, Fran?"

She looked at me with a playful smile. "Are you proposing to me?"

"I guess I am."

And that's how it happened.

We were married in Billy and Janice's apartment on December 26th, 1976. No tux, no band, no limos. A stoned-out Rabbi who drove up in a VW bus with a portable chupa.

The rest, as they say, is history.

Chapter Sixteen
Homeward Bound

Walter, a member of Dr. Trento's staff, patiently ran down a list of guidelines with Fran and me before discharging me from the hospital. He began by presenting a list of numerous prescriptions that would have to be filled. He then handed Fran a small vial of a mild hand soap to be used to clean my incision on a daily basis to prevent infection. He instructed me to avoid lifting anything over ten pounds, pushing, pulling, or doing vigorous arm exercises. My severed breastbone was held together with wire and would need three months to mend. He cautioned me to stick to a "Healthy Heart" diet, low in fat and cholesterol. Be especially aware of salt intake. It was essential to completely avoid very salty foods and never add it for taste, as I so often did. My level of activity should be gradually increased daily.

Walter recommended to begin my recovery with two to three ten minute walks each day, then add two minutes to the walks to build up my stamina. The goal was twenty minutes three times a day on flat ground. In six weeks' time, I should try to walk an hour a day for a total of three miles. I would then be able to start most activities, including driving and travel. Until that time, I would have to be a passenger, as long as I wore a seat belt and took a break every hour if the drives were long.

Control of my blood pressure was extremely important. I needed to measure it every morning before taking my meds and again before dinner. I mentioned that our bedroom was on the second floor and asked if it was okay to climb the staircase. We could set up a bed in our downstairs den if it wasn't. To my relief, he said it would be fine. Just take a few steps at a time, pause, and then continue.

"And speaking of the bedroom..." I said playfully, smiling at Fran.

"Everyone responds differently. You'll know. It's usually three to four weeks, when you're able to walk two miles without feeling short of breath or tired. Anything else?"

"I think you've covered everything."

"Dr. Trento will see you in the office to remove the stitches and monitor your new valve a week from Wednesday. But, if for some reason you're not feeling well, the incision doesn't look right, anything at all, don't hesitate to call. We're always there for you."

"Thanks for everything, Walter. Everyone from your office has been great."

"Glad to hear it. Just be patient, don't rush anything, and you'll be fine. Okay?"

"Fran will make sure of that."

Fran checked the closet and drawers of my night stand to make sure we weren't leaving anything behind. Within a few minutes, an aide had entered the room and eased me into a wheelchair. The coast was cleared for takeoff, and we made our exit. I smiled at the day nurse as the aide wheeled me past her station. She wished me well and said goodbye. I was silently pleased with myself, like a proud senior who had just received his diploma on graduation day.

As we continued on, I turned and looked out at the members of the hospital staff busily going about their jobs, seeing to needy patients, monitoring their computers. I suddenly noticed the tall, black attendant, wearing his signature hairnet, emerge from a room across the hall. He was quietly going about his job, delivering his lunch trays with his signature phrase of good will, "Enjoy your meal." Our eyes met. I waved goodbye. He smiled broadly and gave me the "thumbs up" sign. I nodded my thanks and continued to take my farewell lap.

We reached the elevators in a matter of seconds. The elevators that seemed so many miles away when I began my daily walks had once again become the passageway to the outside world. We reached the street level, and I was in the front lobby once again. I waited patiently with the aide as Fran pulled our silver SUV to the loading area. She opened the passenger door. I cautiously rose from the wheelchair and carefully stepped up into the front seat. I fastened my seatbelt and placed my arm across my chest as a wall of protection.

I was on my way home.

As Fran pulled away from the hospital, I shook my head in disbelief and simply said, "What the hell just happened?"

For the past five days, I had lived in a parallel universe, a self-contained world that had repaired me, nurtured me, and sustained me. I was suddenly cast off into the steady stream of traffic, like a fish that is given a reprieve and thrown back into the river of life. We continued east past the towering Beverly Center and the busy intersection at La Cienega. I looked out at the people going about their lives, entering shops, walking their dogs, sitting at outdoor cafes having lunch.

I felt strangely detached. I was no longer a part of that world, free to move about, drive to my next appointment, or meet friends for dinner at a trendy restaurant. I wondered if those strangers realized how lucky they were. After a couple of miles, we turned left off Beverly Boulevard and drove beneath the shade of the majestic trees that warmed both sides of our lovely block. As we approached the corner, I could make out the sloping green lawn of our front yard.

And then, it appeared before me in all its glory. The beautiful, white palace that has sheltered my family and been our womb for over two decades. It was poised stoically at the top of our driveway, radiating the character of its eighty years. It seemed to be saying "Welcome home." I heard Aabby's familiar bark and spotted her behind the wrought iron gate that enclosed our backyard. I laughed knowingly. This gorgeous dog that was afraid of its own shadow couldn't fool me. I knew her much too well.

I carefully unbuckled my seatbelt and slowly eased my body down to the pavement. I took a breath and started to walk the short distance to the front entryway. Fran anxiously walked beside me, but there was no need to worry. I was more than fine. She reached up and turned off the alarm. I used her arm for support as I climbed the three steps to the front entry. She inserted her key into the lock, turned it to the left, and opened the thick, wood-stained door. I stepped inside and paused briefly. I turned and looked down into our living room.

My eyes gazed out at the expansive, rectangular ceiling bordered on its four sides by giant curved moldings, the rows of family photographs that rested on the glass coffee table in front of our lime green couches, the sleek oak mantel that topped our tiled fireplace, perfectly centered between a pair of matching stained glass windows, the large, curved picture window that dramatically framed the trunks of trees that were entwined like lovers in our front yard.

I was home again. A grateful witness to the sanctuary that Fran and I had lovingly created for the past twenty years. I turned slowly and walked down the hallway towards the kitchen past the colorful oil painting of young dancers that filled the white wall on my left.

Fran wanted to know if I was hungry. She had packed the fridge and the pantry so that she could stay home and keep an eye on me during the first few days. She turned, opened the fridge and began reading off a list of lunch options. I quietly moved behind her and gently placed my hand on her shoulder.

"Frannie..."

She turned around to look at me. I reached out and wrapped my arms around her. We stood for a long moment. She started to turn back towards the fridge. I held her even tighter. I could feel her sigh and relax in my warm embrace. I took a deep breath, stepped back to look at her, and simply said, "Baby, you're the greatest." We kissed.

"Okay, hon, how about a sandwich?"

I sat at the white wood table in our breakfast room and watched Fran prepare lunch. I looked out at our backyard through the glass paneled French doors that led outside. What a cool house, I thought. As we ate our meal, Fran filled me in on messages of good will from family and friends, the latest neighborhood gossip, and went over a list of things to do in the early stages of my recovery.

I suddenly felt tired. All the excitement of the morning, the anticipation, the trip itself, had exhausted me. I slowly rose to my feet, walked back down the hallway and entered our den. I made my way to the black leather couch facing the television and took a seat. I closed my eyes and breathed deeply. My head felt heavy, and my chin dropped to the top of my chest.

It was almost three-thirty in the afternoon when I awoke from my nap. I had slept in a sitting position for almost two hours. I had stored a reservoir of energy and called out to Fran. It was time to take a walk. Fran helped me put on a light jacket.

"Can Aabby come along?" she asked.

"That'd be great," I replied.

We stepped outside in the late afternoon. The February air had a chill to it. We made our way down the driveway. I looked up at the wind blowing through the limbs of trees overhead. I held my head high and looked straight ahead. I took a deep breath and tried to expand my ribcage. Didn't get very far. I tried again and consciously called on my diaphragm for support, like I did when I sang. It was a slight improvement. I had a lot of work to do.

But that was okay. I was on my feet, walking down my block, past the homes of my neighbors. I was outdoors, on a sunny, breezy afternoon, not some sterile, fluorescent hospital corridor. We had passed just four houses when the clock on our cellphone informed us that five minutes had elapsed. I stopped to get a second wind and slowly turned around.

We headed back patiently. I wasn't in a race. As Fran led me up the driveway, I could feel the added strain of walking up an incline. Boy, was I weak. We finally made it. Fran gave me a high-five. I could do this thing. Once safely inside the house, I continued walking through the kitchen and opened the door in our utility room that led to the backyard.

I heard the soothing sound of rushing water and looked out to see the small waterfall that emptied into our koi pond. It called out to me like a muse. I followed it. I took a seat at the stone bench that overlooked the flowing water and gazed down at my large, colorful Zen masters gliding through their water world. A sense of calm washed over me. This had always been my place to meditate. Whenever I was dealing with the daily stress of producing a show, I always found relief in this very spot. It was a magical place where I could heal my spirit. It was working its magic again.

I looked around and admired the pair of sculptured mushrooms I carried in my own two hands and embedded firmly in the soil beneath the giant melaleuca tree, the gripping ficus that coats the stone walls like green carpet, the dwarf papyrus Fran and I planted together, all bordering this spiritual oasis like a scenic backdrop. I was in my lovely backyard, sitting quietly on a stone bench, inspired by the beauty of my surroundings.

Somehow, that wiry, skinny little kid, who had struggled to put the Sunday newspapers together at the Cozy Nook luncheonette, had managed to survive.

All I can say is, "Thank you."

Epilogue

From the time I was discharged from the hospital, I never felt the need to take any pain medication. Occasionally, I would take a couple of Tylenol, but that was the extent of it. That amazed me. By the end of my first week home, I was taking two twenty-minute walks a day. By the end of my second week of recovery, I was eating out at nearby restaurants.

I began cardio-rehab four weeks after the operation. I went for supervised workouts twice a week. By the second week of rehab, I was walking vigorously for twenty-five minutes on the treadmill and riding an exercise bike for an additional twenty minutes.

I began driving on my own after six weeks.

At the end of twelve weeks, I played my first round of golf without any pain whatsoever. The burning in my chest that I experienced when I pushed my golf cart up a hill was completely and totally gone.

Coincidentally, just weeks after my surgery, aortic valve replacement surgery was suddenly front-page news. Former First Lady Barbara Bush, 83, had her aortic valve replaced at the Methodist Hospital in Houston, actor/comedian Robin Williams, 57, had his aortic valve replaced at The Cleveland Clinic and baseball player, Aaron Boone, 36, had his aortic valve replaced at the Stanford University Medical Center. Aaron's situation was exactly like mine. He was born with an abnormal bicuspid valve. Six months after his open-heart surgery, Aaron was back in the starting lineup for the Houston Astros.

Anything else? Oh, yeah, I almost forgot. Fran and I just booked our tickets to Italy.

Arrivederci...

Afterword

I just left Dr. Kedan's office after my annual visit to monitor the condition of my new aortal valve. It has now been seven years since I underwent open heart surgery to replace it. After viewing the results of my echo-cardiogram, Dr. Kedan told me the valve looks like it was put in yesterday.

As I drove home, I couldn't help but think of all the amazing things that I've experienced in the past seven years. Here are just a handful of them:

Fran and I have looked in awe at Michelangelo's David in Florence, stepped inside the Coliseum in Rome, walked among the ruins in Pompeii, and had pizza on the isle of Capri. We've seen a family of bears in Glacier National Park in Montana and hiked in the Alps in Innsbruck Switzerland. Had tapas in Barcelona and drank wine in Provence. In December, we will celebrate my seventieth birthday and our fortieth wedding anniversary in San Miguel de Allende, Mexico.

I wrote my first work of fiction "A Reign Supreme", which was published by Open Road Media.

Through the efforts of my brother Billy, a theatre at his alma mater at NYU Tisch School of the Arts, which was formerly the site of my father's weekend jazz concerts, has been named the Jack Crystal Theatre in his memory.

But the greatest joy of all has been the introduction of six new members of the Crystal tribe. My brother Joel and Barbara's son, Jonathan, and his wife, Vanessa, gave birth to twin girls. Billy and Janice's younger daughter, Lindsay, and her husband, Howie, gave birth to two wonderful boys. And last and certainly not least, our daughter Jackie and her husband Lee have given Fran and me two delightful grandchildren, Coco, now five, and her younger brother, Maxwell Henry, just a year and a half. That's right. Fran and I are grandparents.

I've experienced all this and so much more because of the miracle of modern medicine. Believe me, I take none of this for granted and remain eternally grateful.

Well, that's about all for now. Sorry to run off, but I have a tee time in a little over an hour, and I don't want to be late. I'll be walking the 6 mile course and pushing my cart along the way. It looks like it's going to be a beautiful day.

Acknowledgments

The publication of this book is due to the encouragement of my cardiologist Dr. Ilan Kedan of the Cedars-Sinai Medical Center in Los Angeles who enlightened me to the positive contribution my story could make in helping those contemplating open heart surgery find the comfort to face their fears. To THE Dr. Alfredo Trento, my gifted surgeon who healed my aching heart and his entire team who held my hand through recovery. Special thanks to Dr. Mehmet Oz for spreading the news and Carla Gardini, Donna O'Sullivan and James Avenell for making sure he did. To publicist Cindi Berger for bringing my book to the attention of Barbara Walters, a fellow traveler who faced the same challenge as myself and knew first-hand what I was writing about. The amazing Dr. Robert Klapper for his enthusiasm, support and friendship and Joey Josephs, a talented photographer and lifelong friend from my hometown of Long Beach who helped to make some beaten up photographs come to life. A special thanks to Deborah Morales who wholeheartedly supported this endeavor and to Kareem Abdul Jabbar and our friendship that has endured over half a century. His willingness to contribute his beautifully written and heartfelt foreword is a gift I can never repay. His legendary achievements on the basketball court are only surpassed by his humanity.

To the authors of "You're Nearer," composer Richard Rodgers and lyricist Lorenz Hart for providing me the strength to overcome my grief and bid my mother a final goodbye.

A special vote of thanks to my dear friend and agent Joel Gotler who always believed in my story and made sure it found a safe home in the hands of Tracy Ertl at TitleTown Publishing in Green Bay, Wisconsin. Her passion and enthusiasm is only surpassed by her generosity of spirit. She chose wisely in enlisting the invaluable help of editor Kylie Shannon in making sure my words rang true and the keen artistic eye of Erika Block who brought a touch of class to the interior design.

My heart surgery made me confront my mortality and reminded me to appreciate the miracle and magic of my life – a life that has been defined by the people and things that I love.

And so, I wish to thank those I cherish who inspired me and provided me with a lifetime of memories to fill the pages of this book – my mom and dad, my dear parents who gave me life and shaped my character; my dear brothers who have always had my back; my extended family who have embraced me in their loving acts of kindness and friends too numerous to mention.

To my precious daughter Jackie - I never would have contemplated writing my story if I didn't have a special someone I wanted to tell it to. She, her loving husband Lee and their two delicious children Coco and Max, have enriched my life in ways I cannot measure.

And finally, to my dear wife and soulmate, Frannie Agovino, who on a beautiful summer Saturday morning some forty years ago, stepped off a plane in the Los Angeles Airport, walked into my life and changed it forever.